The buzz about the Barbis

"There are some things in life that you'll never forget. Such for me was meeting the Barbi Twins (well, not everyone is as fortunate as I am!). I met them years ago when I was a segment producer on *Entertainment Tonight*. The segment led to big ratings and a personal relationship with these two wonderful women. Today, I'm the managing editor of *Entertainment Tonight*, and I'm happy to say that I still love the twins, and they still give us <u>BIG</u> ratings!"
—*Glenn Meehan, managing editor and producer of* Entertainment Tonight

"This book is about the secret of recovery: looking good is the result of being healthy. Sia and Shane share with us what their decision to 'go for health' meant to them and document their struggle to achieve spiritual balance and self-acceptance. There is also lots of down-to-earth, practical information and suggestions for anyone suffering from an eating disorder."
—*Joan Mardell, M.A., M.F.C.C, therapist and eating disorder expert*

"One of the things I love most about Shane and Sia is their sense of humor. The fact that they do not take themselves seriously certainly adds to their appeal. I believe their sense of humor has helped them overcome their life obstacles. I love the twins and always enjoy spending time with them."
—*Greg Gorman, internationally-renowned celebrity photographer*

"I remember the first time we ran a story on the Barbi Twins. I could not believe the response: my voicemail was completely full the next day with calls from all around the world. Everyone wanted to know what else the twins were up to. Well, here's your answer—their health and fitness book!"
—*Barry Nugent, producer, E! Entertainment Television*

"'Who are the Barbi Twins, and are they for real?' That's exactly what I thought until I met Shane and Sia in person. Are they for real? Damn right! Should they write a book? You better believe it! Their enthusiasm is unending, and they are as friendly and warm as anyone I know. After spending hours and hours on the phone with them, I feel like we've known each other for years. We are pleased that the Barbi Twins chose *EXTRA* as their foray on the information superhighway, and it's been a first-class ride at 100 m.p.h. ever since."
—*M. J. Roark, producer,* EXTRA

"Shane and Sia Barbi are the most popular international pinups, and they are a source of fascination to men around the world. Now, with this incredible book, they're also a source of inspiration to women. After their honest battle, the remarkable Barbi Twins are the best standard bearers for positive living."
—*Mike Parker, director,* Headline News LA, *former editor of* The Daily Star

"The Barbi Twins are the antithesis of what they appear to be. True, they have all the physical attributes that have made them who they are. But far beyond the obvious, what has astounded me about them has been their knowledge of health, mind and spirit. Their high ratings and marketing make their success self-explanatory."
—Chris DeRose, author of In Your Face and president of Last Chance for Animals

"Wake up; the Barbi Twins are more than meets the eye. Theirs is a story of survivors who have embraced recovery with an openness and honesty that is heroic."
—John Marsh, producer

"Anyone fortunate enough to become close friends with Shane and Sia Barbi—as I have been for the better part of a decade—will discover that under their extraordinary beauty exist two very sharp individuals with gentle souls and giving hearts. Their hands-on study of and experiences with fitness, diet and exercise make them an obvious choice to author a book on women's health."
—Alex Burton, entertainment journalist

"Shane and Sia have been successful and famous print models, but they have also endured the pain and suffering that accompanies eating disorders. Because they have been willing to share their ongoing battle with this disorder, they have enlightened many people about the resources available to them. Their knowledge of food combining and exercise has been of great use to us."
—Candi and Randi Brough, models and "Doublemint Twins"

"Before I read this book, I had never had any contact with the Barbi Twins. I truly enjoyed reading the book. It is an honest, revealing and painful story of two decent and beautiful (inside and out) human beings caught in the trap of Hollywood. I also found the book informative from a nutritional point of view, practical (it includes recipe suggestions), eye-opening for the younger generation and quite helpful as a tool for anyone suffering from overeating, obesity, bulimia, anorexia or any other eating disorder. Last, but not least, I found the book quite uplifting from the standpoint of spirituality and transformation to wholeness. It is a powerful gift to all human beings, especially women and our younger generation. I thank the Barbi Twins for their contribution to the health and well-being of other women. They have proved that brains, beauty and a wonderful humanistic character can really go together."
—Mimi T. Salamat, Ph.D., FAAA, CCC-A, Texas Tech University

dying to be healthy

A BREAKTHROUGH DIET, NUTRITION AND SELF-HELP GUIDE

Sia Barbi

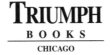

TRIUMPH
BOOKS
CHICAGO

Publisher's Note: Neither this nor any other diet or exercise program should be followed without first consulting a healthcare professional. If you have any special conditions requiring attention, you should consult with your healthcare professional regarding possible modification of the programs contained in this book.

This book is available in quantity at special discounts for your group or organization. For further information, contact:

Triumph Books
601 South LaSalle Street
Suite 500
Chicago, Illinois 60605
(312) 939-3330
Fax (312) 663-3557

Printed in the United States of America

ISBN 1-892049-42-2

Front and back cover photography by Gray Gorman.
Interior photography by Ryan Patterson and Gray Gorman except where indicated otherwise.

Cover design by Eileen Wagner.

Contents

A word of appreciation

Living with Shane Barbi is like joining the army—it's not just a job, it's an adventure! There is never a dull moment living with her, and it would take all of the Smithsonian libraries to describe her. But bottom line is, Shane saved my life. She *is* my life. When we first met, I wasn't attracted to the obvious—her fame and beauty. I was attracted *in spite of* the obvious. I usually stayed away from Hollywood-type women. I've learned some lessons in this town, and I have discovered too many "wannabes" in the disguise of "down-to-earth" girls. Shane was (and is) totally different.

Unlike most infamous or famous people, Shane walked away from the Tinseltown opportunities that most women in her position would kill for. Instant fame was practically dropped in her lap, and I think that hurt her recovery from addiction. We initially bonded because we both shunned Hollywood, yet we could not go out of the house without being pegged. What most consider lucky—being very well known—we felt was stigma. It does not allow you the freedom to live a normal life or associate with everyday people.

I'm glad I never knew Shane's image before we met. To me, she has always been natural and sports loving, and she wants a family much more than a career. She understands that I was an athlete who turned into an actor due to an injury. She saw me as someone who never asked for fame—she saw the real me—and I can reciprocate. We love to have long, deep discussions about theology, philosophy and politics. We learn from each other, respect each other's views, yet usually have a mutual understanding.

Living with a food addict in recovery is much like living with a recovering alcoholic. I never knew that it's really the same disease, only the "drug of choice" is different. We help each other because we both have the same struggles, yet want to progress. Living one day at a time is so much easier when you do it with someone you love, and they understand you completely. I always remember that she was there for me when no one else was, and I will return the favor if it ever becomes necessary.

—*Ken Wahl, actor and husband of Shane Barbi*

Foreword

This book is not a glitzy autobiography about the Barbi Twins and their showbiz pals. Rather, it's a valuable tool. *Dying To Be Healthy* incorporates the twins' inspiring recovery saga with a virtual encyclopedia of healthy living tips that the Barbi Twins don't just preach—they also live. They are painfully aware that fatal eating disorders have become a national epidemic. They've seen the devastation first hand.

Sia and Shane Barbi's famous transition from Malibu beach gals to international celebrities came fast and furious. But they never wanted to be pinups in the first place. Growing up on their daddy's farm in the hills of Malibu, they happily milked goats and drove tractors. And they fantasized about someday becoming athletes, veterinarians, or Catholic *nuns*!

However, the future Hollywood icons grew up in a show biz clan. The Andrews Sisters were their great-aunts and their godmother was the legendary Dusty Springfield. So the convent would have to wait. In between their farming duties, they began modeling (separately) at the age of seven.

After an agent convinced them to pose together in 1990, the resulting Barbi Twins billboard on the Sunset Strip caused fender benders and worldwide press. Hugh Hefner stood up and took notice. And so did everybody else! Their 1991 *Playboy* cover sold out in a couple of weeks. Their second *Playboy* cover, in 1993, became the best-selling issue in *Playboy* history! One Wall Street signing was so big that it nearly turned into a riot. Even Hef was amazed.

In 1995 Princess Diana caught thirteen-year-old Prince William with some pinup shots of the Barbis. She wrestled them out of Will's grip in front of a sea of reporters and it was covered all over the world press. Scores of Leno and Letterman jokes followed. Pretty soon there were

Barbi Twin references popping up on sit-coms, during *Saturday Night Live*, and in movies. Daytime talk shows found they were getting huge ratings whenever they booked the Barbis and TV producers offered the gals truckloads of money to star in their own series.

Filmmaker Blake Edwards even proposed a sequel to his movie *10*. This time, he said, it would star the Barbis and be called *20*. But the girls told Hollywood to take a hike. "We can't act!" they insisted quite candidly.

It was that brutal honesty in such a phony business that caused *Wiseguy* star Ken Wahl to fall in love with Shane Barbi. They married in 1997 and moved into a Malibu beach house. While sister-in-law Sia says Ken is terrific, she swears that when she settles down some day it will be with a simple cowboy rather than a famous playboy.

By this point the twins were appearing in huge spreads in European fashion magazines and on runways. A Topps comic book featuring crime-fighting Barbis sold like hotcakes. It seemed a Hollywood dream had come true and the girls had it all. But secretly, Sia had been in and out of hospitals so often as a result of severe bulimia that doctors told her she was about to die. During that low period, the Barbi Twins had a horse and a whole race named after them at Hollywood Park. But Shane says that if she and Sia had been horses themselves, they surely would have been taken out of their misery.

That's when the twins, at the height of their fame, shocked their showbiz pals. Despite TV and movie offers from all corners, they took a sabbatical to focus on their recovery, devouring information on health. Both got degrees in nutrition. They started to feel that instead of just looking pretty to get attention, they were *earning* it with hard work.

A recent *New York Post* feature and a *USA Today* cover story show the Barbis reaching out to women as respected eating disorder spokespersons. And happily, women are listening! The twins, who were once dismissed by some as Hollywood bimbos, are now lecturing to standing-room-only crowds at universities and high schools across the country. They're debating some of the country's top doctors on matters of nutrition and health. Even *48 Hours* and *E! True Hollywood Stories* tagged along to document the amazing new Barbis-in-recovery phenomenon. Crowds lined up to hear the Barbis teach at Learning Annex centers. And a made-for-television Barbi movie is also being developed.

The twins have often been compared to Erin Brockovich, who also mixed beauty with brains. With this book, they prove you should never judge a Barbi by her cover!

—*Pete Trujillo, noted entertainment reporter*
Los Angeles, California
March 2001

Chapter 1
From the heart
(by Shane and Sia)

When we were asked to write this book, we originally planned to include only health and nutrition information. We quickly realized, though, that those topics are only part of our story. We decided that to truly help people, we would have to share some dark and painful truths about our past food addictions, our bulimia and our subsequent recovery. For us, recovery has become the vital turning point in our lives, and this book could not be written without including our search for wisdom and peace.

Please note: Neither our publishers nor we endorse, in any way, a specific twelve-step program or diet institution. Neither do we endorse a particular religion or individual philosophy.

Instead, this book represents our life experiences, personal research and our hopes and prayers that you may gain inspiration and strength from our excruciating mistakes. You, too, can live healthfully and happily, and free from fear and addiction. We hope this book will help. In fact, we are counting on it.

— *Shane and Sia*

Sia Barbi:

My sister and I are adult children of alcoholics. Unlike a co-dependent spouse or Alanon member who may eventually decide to walk away from a negative home situation, we never had a choice. Although we caught glimpses of familial normalcy from the lives of our childhood friends and from watching television (so, unlike what we had in our family), we, nevertheless, believed that we lived a fairly average lifestyle.

But we grew up learning how to keep secrets. From the time we were toddlers, Shane and I hid behind shame and guilt, living constantly with the fear of being abandoned. We learned not to trust anybody but each other. We started out as victims and continued to play those roles until recovery showed us amazing new possibilities. Do I wish I had a normal upbringing? That is like asking if I enjoy being a twin. How would I ever know otherwise?

Interestingly, our lowest personal period actually came in the middle of our commercial success in 1991. Our Hollywood billboard on the Sunset and La Cienega intersection was drawing daily crowds—it even caused traffic accidents! Although we made the cover of the *LA Times*, published a lucrative calendar and posed for Playboy, none of that mattered to us. In fact, we did not want our friends and family to discover our newfound fame because we were slightly embarrassed. We realized that some people would think the publicity was silly and exploitive—and we were ambivalent about success anyway. It was hard to be naked in front of cameras when we felt unattractive almost all the time.

Sudden fame actually made us revert deeper into isolation and eating disorder, which my sister and I had shared since age seven. In the beginning of the media uproar, we refused press phone calls and interviews altogether. And yet, this mystique put us in even more demand. Everyone was asking, "Why would the famous sisters suddenly turn down million-dollar offers and countless film opportunities?" Why indeed?

Shane and I were like drug addicts—we felt constant shame, guilt and fear. Our carefully packaged new images turned our lives into a Cinderella story, but we knew the clock would strike midnight very, very soon. What good would all of that money do if we only spent it on fancy binge foods and decadent fat farms? Fame would expose how insecure and sick we were. It felt like hanging our dirty underwear out on the Goodyear blimp.

We decided to go on a "sabbatical" which lasted almost five years. We concentrated on recovery and focused on developing skills in other areas, such as our own health and well-being. Yet, during this time, the press still hounded us.

Then, Shane's marriage to Emmy-award winning actor Ken Wahl (from CBS's WISEGUY) utterly blew our camouflage. Shane and her new husband Ken (star in films like *The Warriors, Fort Apache, The Bronx and The Favor* with Brad Pitt) made the cover of every tabloid in town with the sickening headline "Ken and Barbi Wed." So,we unwillingly landed in the spotlight once again. (While Ken is a talented actor, he thankfully chose to bow out of the Hollywood scene altogether. This, of course, suits us perfectly—what a relief.)

Others might find this type of fame flattering, but to us it is horrifying. When you are battling a disease that robs you of confidence, self-esteem and strength, you lose the desire for any true success or benevolence. Believe it or not, we never believed in our potential for fame...we lived our disease every single day. There was no room for anything else.

I really want to "come out of the closet" with this book. It is not your typical diet tale, but nothing we do is ever typical. We have already posed naked, so now we are prepared to bear our souls, and that's so much harder to do! I want to educate our readers, but most of all, I want to share hope. Hope is the beginning of fulfilling all your dreams.

Shane Barbi:

Food and fitness have been our obsession, our career, our life and almost our death. We started modeling at the age of seven. We immediately became body-obsessive and learned how to self-medicate with our drug of choice: food.

As kids, we were always educational over-achievers, so it is ironic that we first became famous as pin-ups. Modeling in our teens was like playing Superman: the geeky guy gets dressed up for special occasions, flies out of a phone booth, accomplishes miracles, then dashes back into that secret hiding place in the booth. Modeling was such a small part of our lives, and that phone booth got very lonely.

Now our terrifying experiences have a higher purpose. I'd like our readers to know that we have been advised not to announce our battle with bulimia, or write about it. We were told, "What man would buy a calendar or a centerfold of a woman who sticks her fingers down her throat?" Not a pretty fantasy! That's too bad, because we know we also have an audience who is sick of picture-perfect, unrealistic models who seem to never suffer the indignities of real life. We suffer; you suffer (who does not suffer?), and it's time to acknowledge that.

I'd like to believe that there are no mistakes in life, and no co-incidences, either. There is a purpose to everything. Naturally, you can blame your alcoholic family, the sexist media, or the donut in front of you for your unhappiness. That is your choice. We have chosen, however, to seek absolution and to share our obsessions with our audience and loyal fans.

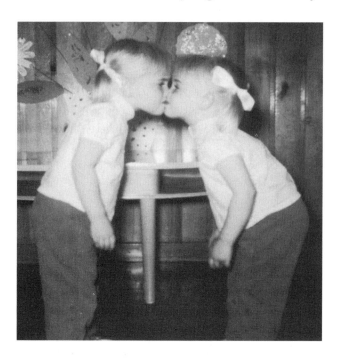

Shane and Sia as little girls

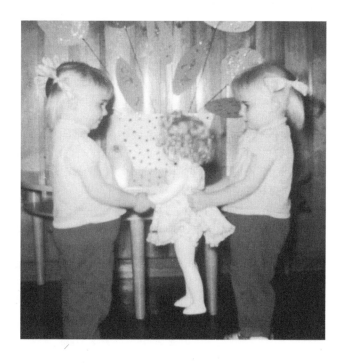

We are not excusing or justifying our actions in any way. In fact, if we could impart a single message, it would be to tell you to achieve your dreams with focus and discipline. You can start on this incredible journey by learning the Serenity Prayer:

"God grant me the serenity to accept the things I cannot change, the courage to change the things I can, and the wisdom to know the difference." There is a difference between giving up and surrendering. If we do the footwork, if we do not give up, yet surrender to the Higher Power, it will lead us to where we are supposed to go.

The Awakening

After 20 years of food abuse, we realized that our diet tricks were making us heavier, and then they stopped working altogether. Recovery began to signify not only abstaining from bingeing or purging, but also making amends, attempting full honesty and transforming our lives into a journey of redemption and hope.

One of our most poignant turning points came in spring 1996 when I overdosed on laxatives. We had been experimenting for almost two years, gaining higher tolerances for more and more prescription and over-the-counter diet aid varieties. Somewhere along the line, we decided that throwing up every day was hard work, and that laxatives were the magic bullets to eternal thinness and happiness.

On that one night, we timed our consumption—as usual—so we would not need the bathroom at the same time. After you take a tremendous dose of laxatives, you usually need to run—not walk—to the bathroom within the hour. For the next forty minutes or so, stomach cramps and painful diarrhea double you over. Even as you feel the huge spasms pass through your intestines, you feel stoned, very relieved and sort of excited to lose the weight (we would lose up to 10 unhealthy pounds of food, bile and water, all at once).

When you overdose on laxatives, as I did that fateful night, diarrhea is usually followed by excruciating vomiting since you have, essentially, poisoned yourself. As my sister tells it, I flailed and fell to the floor with dry heaves; foam began spilling and frothing from my mouth. When I lapsed into unconsciousness, Shane cried, screamed and paced for a few minutes as these thoughts flew through her head, "Who should I call? Will they tell the tabloids? Is my sister dying?"

To Shane, it felt like a million years before the paramedics took me away to establish an IV to replace the electrolytes and water I had violently lost. As a food addict, you push the envelope every day, but this was different: I had taken the equivalent of 100 laxatives. Just for a moment, close your eyes and picture your own sister or best friend collapsing on the floor with bloody froth flowing out of her mouth and calling out to you in desperate pain. The image stays with you forever.

Right after I almost died, we learned to commit and surrender to our obsessions. Then we really jumped into the twelve-step programs, therapy, workshops, church and meditation. Our recovery saved our lives. In a strange way, we were lucky to grow up in and around Alcoholic Anonymous. We knew recovering alcoholics who underwent remarkable transformations with spiritual guidance. When our lives spun so completely out of control, we were forced to make the ultimate choice. Continue being addicted to food, which might kill us? Or choose to have a healthy recovery and work toward serenity? And would we know sanity and serenity if we met them head-on? Hmmm.

Recovery is about lifting the obsessions of the body (and the ego) and putting energy into contribution, especially anonymously. Now true success for us is helping other people. We still have our struggles, find daily reprieve from our obsession and continually strive for progress, not perfection. We must often be reminded that sainthood is not bestowed on the living. We hope our stories provide inspiration.

We have learned that miracles exist. We are very grateful to be alive.

Scary diet stories

Our tales of dieting horror are not entertainment. Bulimia is serious, powerful, cunning and baffling. Our stories may appear funny, but then some of you will identify with the insane things we did, and that is why we represent them this way. Whether you have chosen drugs, alcohol or food as your obsession, all addictions distort common sense and create perpetuate denial.

If you find yourself getting hungry as you read any of these stories, put down the book immediately and take a brisk walk around the block!!!!

Scary diet story 1

Even when we were children, our food disorder was active, despite the fact that we were skinny little twigs. We even joined the Girl Scouts to get closer to the Girl Scout cookies!! Forget sewing badges and tying knots; those cookies were worth wearing the goofy green outfits.

We had originally planned on selling the cookies and eating just some of our profits. We had hoped to still earn earning enough money to take the scout trip to Disneyland. Amazingly, however, over the course of a week, we ate the profits, the net, the gross, the bonuses—everything. Between the two of us, we ate 20 cases of cookies! Forget Disneyland; we were going to do hard time, Girl Scout-style.

And it was at about just the same time that the opportunity to model came knocking. We needed to repay the cash—and fast. Interesting that this event was the birth of our disease AND of our modeling careers.

Scary diet story 2

As children, we were creative and artistic. Those skills came in exceptionally handy when it came time to camouflage food: according to our family, we could make a cake look exactly the same size after consuming nearly half of it. We would remold the cake, making it smaller and rounder and smear the frosting on thinner. We also became exceptionally good at creating alibis when food and sweets were missing at home.

No matter how our mother intercepted us, begged and reasoned with us to stop bingeing, we only became more cunning and manipulative. Although our mom knew something terrible was happening, she could not help us. One year, when we were still very young, our mother was given a big, beautiful box of chocolates as a Christmas gift. She carefully hid it in one of our favorite holding areas: her closet (sucker.) Dismantling the gift-wrapped masterpiece felt like *Mission Impossible*: We almost had to assign each piece a number to place it back correctly. We still recall how those little chocolates glistened in the dim closet light. It was as though they were shouting, "Eat me, try me, taste me."

The first step was to carefully remove the overcrowded inner section of the chocolates. The circumference would have to come in just a bit. If we ate the bottoms, we could make it look like they actually melted through the wrappers. No wrappers—no evidence. Well, at the end of this extravaganza, one little treat was left. Oops. Needless to say, the next day our hearts dropped when there was a lock on our mother's closet. I guess she could be a sucker only so many times. When she stopped keeping food at home, we just bought it ourselves.

Scary diet story 3

Like with millions of other young teens, puberty did a number on our circumference. We became completely obsessed with food and with getting rid of our budding curves. Even our after-school baby-sitting efforts became opportunities to eat. It was not simply the taste of the mashed banana or split pea soup that joyously beckoned. Even the way those perfect little jar tops would click open was exciting to us. Our Pavlovian response kicked in early—and stayed put for the next 20 years!

One particular baby-sitting incident stands out in my memory. A neighbor asked me to baby-sit her toddler one Monday evening. Ecstasy! I still remember the menu: blended apricots and pears, plus a vegetable bean mixture that tasted like dip.

As I fed the baby dinner, the ratio suddenly became: two bites for you and one for me; one bite for you and one for me. I played the game endlessly; the spoon turned airplane flying to my mouth. He eventually stopped eating and just watched me gobble up his dinner.

I am sure that if his parents had hidden a video camera, I could have been arrested for child neglect or endangerment. Teaching a baby what bulimia looks like is unforgivable.

Chapter 2

Diets: from fasting to food fads

The word "diet" alone sells—without any proof, research or common sense. In this country, "diet" is usually a euphemism for quick fix, and the less we have to work at weight loss, the more a product or diet plan sells. Strictly for the purposes of this book, we categorize diets into these groups:

- *Protein diets or Low-carbohydrate diets*
- *High-carbohydrate diets*
- *All-you-can-eat diets*
- *Gimmicks (some may work, some are just plain ridiculous)*
- *Fasting, Cleansing diets, Starvation or Very-low-calorie diets*
- *Miscellaneous diets*

TO OUR READERS: Please, note that the descriptions of these popular food plans are our personal interpretations, or the way in which we practiced them. Always check with your doctor!

Protein diets

There are cycles of popularity attached to these trendy food plans. Ten years ago (as well as today), protein diets were popular because of the large amount of fat calories and the often-unlimited amounts of protein you were "allowed" to eat during the program. Protein plans, like the ever-popular *Zone Diet*, commonly claim that the hormone insulin is the culprit in gaining weight.

In a nutshell, if blood delivers more glucose (the body's main source of fuel from breaking down the foods we eat) than the body needs, the hormone insulin signals the liver and muscles to take up the surplus. When blood glucose is too high—and muscles are not using this fuel for activities such as exercise—the body corrects itself by siphoning off the excess to the liver (to be stored as future fuel), or it converts it to fat.

Most high-protein diets are based on the premise that if you eat a big carbohydrate-packed meal and do not use those future glucose calories as fuel, the pancreas over-secretes insulin, driving glucose, too quickly, into cells. When those glucose stores are filled to capacity, the liver breaks down the extra energy molecules and handily stores them as fat. And fat cells can store unlimited amounts of fat. But here is the rub: The body stores all incoming excess calories as fat—even those extra calories from protein and dietary fat. So why avoid carbs in moderate, digestible portions?

Incidentally, high-protein diets also result in high intake of cholesterol since they are usually high in animal fat. Very-high-protein diets may also cause fatigue since the liver and other body processes are working overtime.

Liquid-only protein diets went out of style when they started killing people (or damaging their kidneys). Other popular protein diets are the *Scarsdale Diet, Atkin's Diet* and *Stillman Diet*. (We personally consider the *Zone* a more balanced version, but many nutrition experts do classify the *Zone* as a very-high-protein diet.)

It is also important to remember that eating higher amounts of protein—whatever the reason—is harmful. If a bodybuilder, for instance, consumes high quantities of protein, it would not help him grow more muscle, as there is a limit to how much protein the body can turn into muscle at a given time. Excercise makes you grow—eating more egg whites doesn't. Moreover, our bodies CAN NOT store protein. Excess protein overloads our kidneys by causing excess urination. A recommended dosage for a regular person (bodybuilders shoud consume a little more) is, in grams, 1/2 of our body weight in pounds.

High-carbohydrate diets

High-carbohydrate diets tend to be lower in fat and protein. Frequently recommended by nutritionists, they are often moderate and well-balanced, incorporating all the food groups. Carbohydrates, however, hold nine times more water than protein or fat grams, so women who tend to have edema (water retention), might think added water weight from carb-rich diets is actually fat weight—it is not, but it is frustrating, nonetheless. Just remember: eating too much of anything can cause weight gain—and fat storage. Popular high-carb diets include the *Longevity Diet, Pritikin,*

Macrobiotics and Durhan Diets.

The classic *Pyramid Food Chart* is usually the gold-standard curriculum in nutrition schools, and it is a high-carb food program. It recommends you get most of your daily calories from complex carbohydrates (grains, legumes, and cereals), fewer calories from proteins (dairy, poultry, meat) and the least amount from fat (oils, butter, sweets).

All-you-can-eat diets

These diets are understandably, some of the most popular food plans around. On the *Beverly Hills Diet* or even *Dr. Heller's Diet* (associated with Richard Simmons) guidelines state that during certain times of day, you can eat anything you want in unlimited quantities. But these diets also severely limit caloric intake for the rest of the day. While they might seem to work at the onset, it may be because you are shocking your digestive system and eating fewer calories per day. Lack of carb calories will leech more water from your body, causing an immediate—but temporary—water-weight loss.

Gimmick diets

These include anything—counting how many bites it takes to chew, subscribing to the *Cabbage Soup Diet*, nibbling a grapefruit before meals, or repeating prayers or affirmations before you eat. Since everybody reacts differently to specific diets, how can one magical crystal, voodoo doll or mantra help everyone? If it did, why don't we all just do it to lose weight once and for all?

There is another classic diet gimmick: one hour before a regular carb-rich meal (like pasta or a sandwich) eat a tiny, fattening snack (like a truffle). Some devotees claim that eating this decadent treat prior to any meal helps the body feel satiated and trips your brain transmitters to make you feel already full.

We actually like the prayer-affirmation diet theory (a pseudo-gimmick). Giving your food to God first is a step towards resisting out-of-control bingeing. Some research has shown that stress actually interferes with efficient digestion and many create toxins in your digestive system.

Positive mantras train you to chew slowly, to be aware of your food, and to avoid over-eating. Being grateful for a delicious meal also inspires you to maintain a healthy diet regimen.

Carbohydrate loading: The expression "carbohydrate loading" is a term used by athletes who use fuel-regulating foods before a sporting event in order to maximize energy and athletic performance. Carb-loading supposedly does this by tricking the body into storing extra fuel before a competitive event. While it is not exactly a diet gimmick, consuming larger-than-normal amounts of carbohydrates during the days or weeks leading up to a special athletic event, like a marathon, can help sustain energy levels. An example of improper loading is using a high-carb regimen and supplementing it with drugs, caffeine or natural enhancers like creatine or human growth hormone.

Carbohydrate loading can often have negative side effects that outweigh any performance advantage, including weight gain, swollen muscles, edema and abnormal heartbeat. Also, the average eater (or dieter) does not need the huge amounts of calories pro athletes need.

Gimmick diets tend to stress nutritional imbalance by emphasizing one food or food group. Other examples of what we consider gimmick diets are: the *Cabbage Soup Diet*, the *Lecithin-Kelp-Vinegar-B6 Diet*, the *Candy Diet*, the *Grapefruit Diet*, etc.

[*NOTE TO OUR READERS*: There are several popular rice diets, including one practiced at a famous East Coast institute, which healthfully starts out with a simple, low-cal carbohydrates, mostly incorporating rice. In a more balanced way, the institute then slowly adds lean chicken, fish and other proteins and fats which eventually balance and complete the food plan. That one is the best of the bunch, and not truly a "gimmick."]

High-fat diets

These diets are unreliable, unbalanced and dangerous, especially if they include many saturated fats (which clog your arteries and may lead to high blood pressure and heart disease). High-fat food plans try to "trick" your metabolism by limiting normal amounts of carbohydrates. Over time, high-fat diets will tax your liver and kidneys, cause weight gain and stress your body.

Fasting, cleansing, or very-low-calorie diets

The definition of fasting is "food abstinence." Scary! There are many interpretations of fasting, ranging from drinking only distilled or drinking water and fruit juices to omitting entire food groups. Very-low-cal diets or liquid-fast diets vary anywhere from 300 to 800 calories. (A calorie, by the way, is a unit of energy gleaned from the foods we eat.)

Low-calorie diets (as opposed to very-low-calorie diets) can boost health and immune system; invigorate your body and mind. The trick is to make sure that the diet is balanced, and that all nutrients are present. It has been discovered that a nutritional plan with a caloric count slightly lower than that a person would optimally need, actually strengthens the body and slows down the aging process. Such low-calorie dieting is especially beneficial at an old age. Low-calorie and wholesome food is also crucial for preventing cancer, as cancer is caused by nutritional imbalance (and environmental pollution), rather than by genetic predesposition. Remember, to be healthy and fit you do not need to overstuff your stomach.

Fasting can provide quick results in a short amount of time, but at the expense of your health. Bottom line: limit fasting to less than two days unless you do it under a doctor's supervision. Interestingly, when animals are sick, they often do not eat solid food for a day or so until the problem corrects itself. Maybe, humans can imitate that lesson; but when people fast repeatedly, it cripples the metabolism and prevents the feelings of well-being and self-confidence.

When you chronically fast or eat minimal calories in the quest to quickly drop pounds, an unfortunate thing happens: fasting lowers your controversial "set point," the point at which your body wants to settle unnaturally, and where it feels most comfortable in weight, regardless of aesthetics. We have found that during most moderate diets, you tend to discover this plateau generally at the three-week mark. Some experts consider this to be your "natural" set point, the weight at which your body refuses to drop more weight.

To blast past a frustrating set point, many experts believe that you must first eat more calories—and higher quality foods—as well as increase your activity level and exercise goals. (It means a lot of hard work, which never sounds as appetizing as the quick fix.)

Any diet under 1,200 calories is almost guaranteed to be unbalanced and nutrient-deficient. Anything under 800 calories is classified as a Very-low-calorie diet—and you are just asking for trouble. Most Very-low-cal plans are unbalanced, unhealthy and necessitate nutritional supplements and/or supervision.

When someone eats under 800 calories or so per day, a phenomenon occurs, called ketosis, whereby the body uses fat without the help of carbohydrates. Ketones are unwanted and abnormal cellular biochemicals, which are made only when the body does not have available fuel sources, namely carbohydrates. Ketosis makes dramatic and quick weight loss possible—but the deficiency is temporary and due to the lack of cellular water. This is a dangerous state for your body. Ketosis causes excessive urination (which contributes to additional dehydration), feelings of light-headedness, halitosis and nausea. Ketosis during pregnancy causes mental retardation in infants.

Interestingly, body weight has nothing to do with the time limit or endurance of a successful fast. A thin person who prepares herself for the rigors of fast, by eating simple raw foods and juices, will have fewer crises. (Researchers usually classify a fasting crisis as anything from dizziness to severe cramps and vomiting). On the other hand, an overweight junk food addict who also indulges in coffee, chemicals and a stressful lifestyle may not be able to endure a fast for any extended amount of time.

In most cases, a fast should be carefully broken by eating one fruit every two hours, six times during the first day. Once you have lost a lot of weight through unhealthy ketosis, however, do not expect to lose much weight on another diet in the future. Your body will resist, and your metabolism will suffer greatly.

Hygienic diet

Hygienic is a term coined by fasting gurus that means raw or perfect food combinations. We followed a hygienic diet for a few years and had fairly good results until unhealthy side effects surfaced. We provide it for your curiosity only. Do not combine fruit with another food. Do not combine, in one meal, fruit from different fruit categories. The four fruit categories are:

- *Sweet: bananas, dried fruit, grapes*
- *Sub-acid: apples, pears, peaches*
- *Citrus: pineapple, oranges, lemons, berries*
- *Melons: melons best served without ANY other fruit*

Vegetables: Eat alone or only with proteins. (Eat raw seeds and avocado with vegetables only). We ate two meals a day consisting of two different kinds of fruit, in the morning. Then, at night, we consumed seeds or avocado with a ton of raw vegetables. The fat content of nuts, seeds and avocado did not matter because of the small amount of food we ate and its wholesome quality. Whether our meals were highly nutritious or not, we were not consuming sufficient calories to sustain us.

Food combination theories

All combo concepts are similar. In theory—and this is a stretch—starches (carbs) and proteins are supposedly metabolized in different areas of our digestive system, and utilize different enzymes. Mixing proteins and fats with carbohydrates may cause starch to rush to the stomach, causing enzymes to malfunction and to slow down digestion, thereby storing additional calories as fat.

In actuality, we sometimes lost pounds on combination and hygienic diets, but much of the weight loss was due to calorie deficits, and our consumption of mostly low-cal , raw fruit and vegetables. However, food combining also prevents dining out, eating most snacks or consuming sufficient protein (we flirted with anemia). When we finally went off these diets and began eating forbidden goodies once again, it felt like we were on drugs. This is a great experience in discipline, but it's not a great (or healthy) diet practice.

Glycemic index and miscellaneous diets

We may soon see the glycemic index listed next to fat grams and calorie intake on food labels everywhere. A glycemic response reflects how fast and how high your blood sugar rises after eating a certain food, and how quickly the body responds by bringing that blood sugar level back to normal. Most people can quickly readjust, but some chronic dieters and most of the obese population may have abnormal carbohydrate metabolism and should avoid many foods with a very high glycemic index, including corn, peas and potatoes.

New research shows that health and body weight are not only affected by calorie and fat content, but also by the type of carbohydrates (glycemics) present. Certain carbohydrates are more quickly absorbed and become more readily available for fuel, hence causing sugar peaks and lows.

Interestingly, some controversial research also indicates that in early prehistoric times, women's bodies craved very high-fat and carbohydrate-rich foods. Supposedly, women needed to store more fat and sugar to survive cooler climates and harsh conditions, and they relied on extra body fat for insulation and childbearing. Men were the hunters who needed more protein, the building blocks for muscle growth.

Rotating or allergy diets

One of the most popular plans today is the "rotating" or allergy diet. The premise is loosely built upon some people's inability to break down certain foods—intolerances or allergies—which manifests in uncomfortable symptoms like fatigue, bloating and weight gain. While there are many ways to do it, you can attempt a rotational plan by avoiding a certain food group for a day—say, rice or dairy—and note if allergy symptoms reappear when you start eating that food group again the next day. On the allergy diet, you keep a food diary, grouping foods by type (dairy, grains, fruit, etc.) and note any changes in physiology. You then maintain a chart depicting your reactions after eating certain types of food.

Food allergies—which affect a very small amount of the population, by the way—may also be caused by stress or poor environment. Our certain family member, who has endured bona fide food allergies for years, became a backyard pharmacist using vitamins and herbs to overcome allergies. Prescription medications either had bad side effects or did not produce lasting results.

Her latest revelation is the enzyme therapy. She purchased carefully formulated combinations (from a professional herbologist) of high potency enzymes such as pancreatic enzyme, amylase, and typsin, which will help metabolize the suspected allergenic foods. The theory is that allergies both cause—and are caused by—poor digestion. These prepackaged enzymes normalize and replace what is needed for normal digestion.

Blood type diets

Blood types are said to play a role in determining specific nutritional needs. Why do some people feel healthier and lose weight on mostly proteins, while some people need more carbs, and others still lose weight and maintain maximal health on equal amounts of both. For example, O-positive blood types allegedly do better on high-protein diets. The Blood type diet theory is new and trendy and is based, very loosely, on evolutionary metamorphosis of nutritional needs. Many people swear by this diet!

The pregnant woman's regimen

Though a mother-to-be should never consider dieting, we realize how traumatic weight gain might be to a pregnant woman who has suffered from disordered eating. Research shows that pregnant women may find best, eating frequent, smaller meals, to keep blood sugar steady and avoid energy dips. Besides, large meals often create nausea and digestive disturbances, which accompanies many pregnancies, especially in the first trimester.

A future mom needs as many vitamins and minerals as she can get during this happy time. Perhaps the biggest diet myth is that during pregnancy a woman needs to eat for two—it just isn't so. A pregnant mother needs only an additional 150 calories per day on top of what she normally eats to supplement her baby's healthy growth. Plus, she should be drinking at least 10 cups of water, avoiding alcohol and caffeine, and eating a wide variety of nutrient-dense foods, such as salads, lean poultry and cooked fish.

Pregnant moms should also avoid sugar substitutes and omit excess salt, which causes water retention and bloating. She should get an adequate intake of vitamins and minerals, especially from the food she eats.

Healthy, pregnant women should also maintain a moderate exercise routine—especially if they were regular gym buffs prior to pregnancy. Healthy muscle tissue will make for an easier birth and recovery, and most experts recommend power walking, swimming and light weight lifting if the mother feels comfortable. (Pregnancy is not the time to take up a new sport, however). Of course, discuss any workouts with your doctor, but consider how exercise can benefit both the mother and the baby: regular workouts reduce stress, allow mother to focus on her own body, lessen tension, decrease lower back pain, and strengthen the muscles needed for labor and delivery.

Healing or energy boost diets

Since we are the ultimate diet consumers, we recognize that fact that we have ruined our metabolism, shot our set point, and ruined any chance of losing weight healthfully on any semblance of a normal food plan. Our radical yo-yo diets have helped us develop low blood sugar, slight anemia, digestive problems, amennorhea (lack of menstrual cycles) and crippled any true love for food we have ever entertained.

Since our metabolisms do need to work more efficiently, and since our bodies do need to heal as much as our minds have, we have intermittently explored many alternative diet aids. While you should check with your doctor, the following have been very helpful to us:

We now take vitamins and minerals regularly, and we have found that vitamin B supplementation aids our energy and metabolism in recommended doses.

When we get the sniffles and feel run-down, we consume echinacea, goldenseal, garlic, zinc, antioxidants and herbal citrus drops to prevent colds and flu. Eucalyptus oil in a vaporizer clears sinuses and aids breathing. When we do succumb to colds and viruses, we eat lightly or nothing solid for a day or two—maximum. Warm fruit and vegetable juices keep us hydrated and provide vitamins without stimulating nausea. We drink tea and eat light crackers to help soak up the stomach acids that cause nausea. We do only low impact exercises—if we do not have a fever. The body craves moderation and balance, and there are no short cuts.

Feeling continually sick or sore is a warning sign to take it easy. Occasionally, making up for a sneaky treat or a missed workout is absolutely fine—we are all human! But if you devote long hours and excessive effort to "work off" those extra calories, your body, mind and soul will eventually pay the price.

Recovery programs

In the *Overeaters Anonymous* program that helped save our lives, there is a twelve-step group program called *HOW* (hopefulness, openness and willingness). It proposes something called *"the Grey Sheet,"* which is a balanced, healthy, low-carbohydrate diet. Low in calories (about 1,000-1,200) *the Grey Sheet* slowly incorporates small amounts of add-on foods and calories each month (usually carbohydrates).

The most compulsive overeaters have a problem with assimilating carbohydrates, counting calories and determining what is "healthy." This diet allows you to stop thinking about the food, and work on improving the quality of your life.

The Grey Sheet diet follows a carefully planned, three-meal program: The meals are nutritiously measured with small but balanced portions. You learn to eat to live, not live to eat, since the emphasis is placed on recovery, not on the diet itself.

We have witnessed a lot of hard work and success at *HOW* because the strategy is powerful and must be taken one brave day at a time. It is not easy. We admire those who surrender, let go and abstain from food obsession.

Some dieters have complained about *HOW*, because long-term participation—with low calories and low carbohydrate intake—has made them suffer a sluggish metabolism and other unhealthy side effects. But, rather than dying from starvation—if nothing else—we believe that this survival food plan gives many people a good kick-start in the right direction.

Other *OA* programs allow you to individualize your own diet plans and abstain from foods that trigger your personal overeating habits. *Overeater's Anonymous diets* also stress that weight will come off if you stop eating compulsively and start working on the rules. We have witnessed life-affirming miracles within organized therapy programs like *OA*!

Permanent, healthy weight loss comes in 1-2 pound increments each week. Slow and steady wins the diet race. Any more is water and/or muscle tissue loss, which makes fat return faster. No one gets fat or thin overnight. It takes time to get educated and develop good habits, but those are the ultimate keys to success. Diet Lotto just doesn't exist—work hard now or pay later. Dieting is ineffective, unless it is moderate. Any diet which promises quick results will make the body go into shock—with the inevitable metabolism slow-down. This is also true with overeating: if you suffer from it, take it slow. Do not become "perfect" overnight. As with any addiction, recovery works only when it is gradual. No cold-turkeying!

Balanced, rational and supervised diets

These include *Weight Watchers, Jenny Craig and Sweat Masters* nutritional programs. Meal replacement drinks may help you lose weight, but should not substitute solid nutrition.

We'd like to mention that the *Weight Watcher's* programs tend to be difficult for people with disordered eating because there is such and emphasis on a point system. The dieter must constantly calculate calories, fiber and fat grams. Each type of food has a certain amount of points assigned to it, and according to your weight, you are allowed only so many points. Although *Weight Watcher's* is successful on many levels, we personally believe that it is a difficult plan for obsessive dieters to sustain.

Of course, no diet will do any good if you return to harmful eating patterns. At some point, you must address what made you put on extra weight in the first place. We believe that our grandmothers knew more about healthy nutrition than modern diet gurus ever will.

Perhaps we are not all meant to be vegetarians, yet many people achieve dietary success with legume/grain-based food plans. We have great respect for vegetarians who practice for religious, health or human reasons. We were vegetarians for quite a few years until we became severely anemic from bulimia—and returning to protein consumption from animal sources helped cure this debilitating condition.

Today, we eat small amounts of fish and chicken, but prefer tofu, yogurt, nuts, beans and avocados as meat substitutes. We find that too much meat makes our eyes dull and our skin dry; we get constipated and irritable.

We think most diets and nutritional plans are outdated. Most of them focus on "quick fixes," and not on long-term solutions. However, the "diet market" expects quick fixes. Dieting and weight control have become an obsession for many Americans. Consider the following statistics:

- *By the age of forty, the typical American woman has been on 20 diets.*
- *Over 20 percent of American 16-year-olds are already chronic dieters.*
- *Fifty five percent of all 8-year-olds have already done "something" to lose weight.*

Through all of our experience and research, we have found a very easy system to make our diet very simple, yet effective and super-healthy. We focus on frequent and balanced small meals packed with equal amounts of protein and carbs, and a bit less than half of those calories in fat.

We no longer make rigid rules. The body changes and has different needs at different times in life. Before or after our morning workout, we tend to eat mostly carbs, like oatmeal and fortified cereals. At night we like light, protein-dominant meals, such as a tofu stir-fry and the occasional piece of grilled fish or skinless poultry. We no longer avoid eating fats like the plague. In fact, we have learned that a small amount of fat in our daily diet helps us feel more satisfied and fulfilled.

Eating right is not hard, but it is different. Humans are creatures of habit who resort to pre-programmed behavioral patterns. Fast food and junk food are escapes and can become addictive. Any addiction will sabotage productivity and your long-term goals.

The obsessive food binge creates a lasting blueprint groove in your brain that makes it much harder to start over. Binges have little to do with will power, control or strength. The food obsession can take over and become ritualistic, even causing blackouts, illness and destruction. Often you notice how far you have fallen into an addiction only when it is almost too late to get out. Food obsessions overtake all desires, needs or common sense.

Scary diet story 4

We thought we had to enlist God in our huge diet attempt in college. Though you may not believe this, we thought 40 days and 40 nights of fasting would get us into sleek, chic shape for upcoming photo shoots.

During a school break, we rented an apartment on the third floor of an apartment complex in Arizona. We begged a loyal, foolhardy friend to lock us into our new apartment from the outside. And into that hellish room, we brought 80 gallons of distilled water and spiritual reading material. And that was all we brought.

For nine whole days, we constantly complained and bitched about the hair-brained idea we hatched. We also spent lots of quality time together and constantly played guessing games about what our unknown neighbors were cooking for dinner. We watched endless cartoons because they were the only programs that did not advertise food—which was absolute torture. Then, we had brainstorm sessions after watching Saturday-morning cartoons.

We tied our bed sheets together on day 10, climbed out of the third floor window and ran to the nearest 7-11. This store had our favorite four food groups: candy, pastry, grease and lard. At the end of the fabulous 7-11 food frenzy, we ate nine days worth of food in one ghoulish hour.

Alka-Seltzer, please!

Chapter 3

Fix your metabolism, the truth about fat

Americans are more obsessed with diets and weight loss than any other culture in the world. In addition to the millions and millions of dollars spent on dieting and nutrition programs, 22.5 million Americans are health club members, and almost $3 billion was spent on home exercise equipment last year alone. So why are Americans heavier than people of almost every other nation?

In what is known as the French Paradox, slimmer French citizens do not deprive themselves of enjoying healthy, fattening foods. Cheese, meat and bread are diet staples. The French don't follow the sort of strict diets we follow here—and they drink wine with almost every meal (100 extra calories per glass!) See the connection?

Muscle weighs more than fat. How can you accurately say, for example, that 50 pounds over your "normal" weight classifies you as obese? I think it is the combination of the extra poundage and weight-related health problems, starting with something as "innocent" as breathing problems, that is obesity. Many factors, such as junk food, excess calories, little movement, drugs, heredity, environment, learned behavior, pregnancy, thyroid problems, allergies and depression can cause a weight problem. Moreover, true morbid obesity, when it is to the point of being health-threatening (and which causes isolation and humiliation), is a deep-seated problem. Physical obesity, which is a result of very slow metabolism, can often only be cured by drugs and/or surgery. Special diet and fitness program complemented by therapy can also help.

Soon we will see that calories do not affect us like we think they do. It is better to eat high-quality, high-calorie, balanced, small-portion meals rather than to starve. Frequent meals speed up the metabolism, and there is plenty of energy. Yet, since the portions are small enough to be digested right away, the food is used, rather than stored. We call high-quality, high-fiber foods "broom foods."

These broom foods work your digestive system like a muscle, but leave quickly. Foods that are an "entertainment" rather than nourishment sit around and leach from your body. Their "snoozing" in your digestive tract causes an insulin imbalance and a hypoglycemic reaction of never feeling full, yet leaving you shaky, light-headed and bloated.

Any movement is good for the metabolism. Yet, we have found that excessive over-exercising is like over-dieting. Your body either tires too much (which pumps the adrenals and causes an insulin imbalance again), or becomes addicted to exercise, needing it in order <u>not</u> to gain weight, rather than using it as a bonus "lift" of the metabolism. Each body is different. But, like a diet, exercise should have balance, moderation and variety, so that the body keeps "on its toes" and does not learn a lazy trick.

Fat does not make fat. Hormonal imbalance does. If you do not eat fat, your body will make it, and worse, hang onto it. This is especially true for women because estrogen is stored in fat. We need fat. Certain good (HDL) fats actually burn up bad (LDL) fats. The best fats are monounsaturated, found in olive oil and avocados, or the essential fatty acids, found in primrose, borrage and black currants. "LDL" means low-density lipoproteins; HDL means high-density lipoproteins.

Obesity is defined as increased body weight due to an excessive accumulation of fat. What a relative definition! Obesity to my sis and me equaled not being able to wear our string bikinis. I always called myself a "closet fatty" because no matter how thin I was, I felt I was "bites" away from obesity. And that can be quite close to the truth when you lose control, and your sanity, through an eating disorder.

Weight charts are not only dated, but much too relative. Muscle weighs more than fat. Moreover, measuring could be inaccurate, especially when wearing those expensive, yet silly, wraps to sweat away inches. How many times did my sis and I use layers of Saran Wrap around our bodies! Sure, we looked sexy wrapped up. That was—until we peeled away our pruney skin. The water-weight loss stayed until we drank water, and our bodies were rehydrated. In any case, we would measure our dehydrated legs and get good results on paper, but the weight loss was temporary and unhealthy.

So if you do not use charts, scales or measuring tapes, how do you determine if you're overweight? One fairly accurate measuring tool, which is popular with athletes and models, involves measuring your body fat percentage. First, you figure out your total fat weight. Then, you take your body weight (for example, 200 lbs.) and divide it into your total fat weight (for example, 20 lbs.) which gives you your body fat percentage (in our example .10 or 10%.) Normal recommended ratios are about 10-13% for men and 15-23%—for women. Athletic trainers push for 6-7% for men and 10-13%—for women. Being below 10%, for women, causes a hormonal imbalance and osteoporosis.

If there are signs of easy bruising, blood in urine or stools, anemia or feeling lethargic, your body fat percentage is very likely too low. So, it really comes down to common sense; let go and be reasonable. If a doctor says you're overweight, then you know you are. Get a second opinion, if necessary. Then write a list of what you want, both in your body and in your life. If a thin, athletic body brings you closer to your goals or future, then losing weight will be easier than that in a situation when you just want to look like some top model. Both your body goals and life goals should be practical and consistent with each other. Your desires and needs should remain on the same level.

To say you want to be thin enough to "catch" a rich man could make any woman anorexic. Being thin should be a "symptom" of healthy eating and living, just as being overweight is a "symptom" of consuming wrong foods and, usually, having some suppressed issues. Then, on your list, write out the advantages of achieving these goals. Write down the sacrifices. Weigh them (no pun intended). When someone has health and priorities as the goal, a diet will not be an obsession. I guarantee that being practical about your body is the best way to stay in shape. It is by far better than chasing a dream of being a picture-perfect model. Remember that eighty five per cent of teenagers think they are fat, when they are not. Ninety two per cent of female athletes have some food disorder.

It is rare for someone to become large by simply loving food. People usually overeat to escape or to "deal" with feelings or issues; at least, this has been our experience. Sometimes the issue we deal with is the perception of being overweight. So, we eat more to deal with this issue. This became a paradox. The solution equals the problem. Why did I have a dozen donuts? ... Because I felt fat. ... What else? Denial can be strong.

Large people, especially women, have to be able to cope with the judgmental and belittling attitudes that society holds towards them. Fashion and media have recently been promoting the druggy, teen-age punk look. You know what our motto was when people said we weren't in style? ... "Good, we will bring it into style." I have seen some very overweight people pass medical exams with flying colors. There are overweight people who are happy and self-assured; they do not let the cruel media or peers destroy their feeling of self-worth. I do believe that if you feel good—you look good. If you look good—you're in style. And you can't fake it. People are more attracted to "large confidence," than to a "wimpy twig." Let a healthy everyday regime bring you to where your body should be. Let your body, not your brain (or quick fix), bring your weight to where it is supposed to be. You do the footwork, and let God take care of the results.

New research shows that obese people almost always have excellent metabolism. Excess eating raises metabolism—unless there is a malfunction with thyroid. Only when an obese individual restricts her food intake—her metabolism slows down. The thyroid is still healthy, but the body becomes more fat-efficient. Each cell demands fat during the duration of such a restriction. Less than 30% to 20% of dieters keep their weight off, in fact, most gain more. New research also unveiled that the hormone leptin, found in fat cells, is responsible for notifying your brain that you are full. This study showed that a large percentage of obese people had this hormone dormant.

A closer look at fat

Believe it or not, we all need a good dose of fat in our diet. Fat is the body's primary storage form for energy, and fat pads around the body surround and cushion our vital organs. Fat under your skin insulates the body against temperature extremes, and some dietary fat enhances the food we eat. But the operative word here is "some."

Eating fat does not automatically make more fat. If you steer completely away from eating fat, your body will hang onto it, anyway. (Remember our scientific starvation theory.) This is especially true for women since the female sex hormone estrogen is stored in fat. Women also carry more flab around for childbearing reasons, and we're far more successful at holding onto fat. (Lucky girls!)

Food fat may end up in fat stores on your body, but first it has to be digested, absorbed and transported to its cellular destinations. And keep in mind that all calories are not created equal: it is far more efficient for you to eat balanced, nutritious, smaller-portion meals, a few times a day, than eating three big ones or, worse, starving yourself. Frequent meal grazing revs up that infamous metabolic rate and provides steady energy throughout the day so you can exercise, eat right, and have the energy to enjoy life. Smaller portions are also more easily digested, so you may be less likely to store any extra calories, which your body doesn't need as fat.

Lipids: Triglycerides and Cholesterol

Every cell has fat-like substances that help control and enhance tissue and blood building, hormone production and nervous system function. Fat (lipids) is composed of building blocks called fatty acids. There are three major categories of fatty acids: saturated, monounsaturated and polyunsaturated. (These classifications are biologically based on the number of hydrogen atoms in the chemical structure of a given fatty acid molecule.)

Triglycerides are food fats and represent 95 percent of all the lipids in the body. They are transported to fat depots—like in muscles or breasts—and stored there. Cholesterol is a soft, waxy substance manufactured in the body and plays an important role in brain and nerve cells. Cholesterol is found in animal-based foods as well as in the human body, and is considered the best predictor of a person's chance of suffering cardiovascular disease. Although high cholesterol usually also means high triglycerides, and vice versa, only high cholesterol is fatal.

Within the body, fats travel around, mixing with the particles called lipoproteins (or, collectively, cholesterol). The two different kinds of lipoproteins are called high-density and low-density lipoproteins (HDL and LDL, respectively). When more protein travels with lipoproteins, the higher the density (HDL) molecules and the lower the risk of heart disease. That's why it's been nicknamed "the good cholesterol." HDL also helps remove residue from the "bad cholesterol," called low-density lipoproteins. LDL transports cholesterol via the bloodstream and may cause hardening of the arteries since it sticks to the arterial walls. Only a minimal amount of LDL is needed in the body, and it's good practice to get your cholesterol checked periodically.

Saturated fats

Saturated and unsaturated fats are found in all food. The difference is that saturated fats—the least healthy kind—are usually solid at room temperature (butter, for example). Unsaturated fats are liquid at room temperature—vegetable oils, for instance. The only exceptions are the saturated fats found in coconut and palm oil, which are also liquid at room temperature. (Chemically speaking, a saturated fatty acid is filled to capacity with hydrogen.) Excess saturated fat clogs arteries and may cause heart disease and obesity. Saturated fats are mostly found in animal products, such as meat and cheese. Since our liver uses saturated fat to manufacture cholesterol, excessive intake of saturated fat raises your "bad LDL" cholesterol, and can—if unchecked—prove deadly.

Monounsaturated fats

A monounsaturated fatty acid has one space (mono) of hydrogen missing on the fatty acid chain, and this tends to make it a healthier fat option. Research shows that the monounsaturated fats found in olive oil, canola oil or grapeseed oil reduce the amount of LDL in the bloodstream. Monos do not cause heart disease the way saturated fats do, and they may even help fight cancer. Other monounsaturated fat sources include peanuts, avocados, olives, and other vegetable and nut oils.

Polyunsaturated fats

If monos are missing one point of saturation on their fatty acid chain, then polyunsaturated fats have two or more points of unsaturation. They are found in oils, such as sunflower, safflower, sesame and flax oil.

Polyunsaturated fat is the chief source of the essential fatty acids necessary for proper cell membrane function and many other metabolic and glandular processes.

The human body can synthesize all fatty acids from the food we eat except for two very important polyunsaturated fats: omega 6 and omega 3. Widely distributed in plant and fish oils, both of these fatty acids serve as raw materials from which the body makes hormone-like substances that regulate many bodily functions, including blood pressure, immune response, blood clotting, inflammation from injury and lipid levels. They are very important fats!

Scary diet story 5

There is nothing more exhausting than bingeing, and having to work it all off by exercising for five, six or seven hours straight. Often, the most difficult part of the equation is finding a "safe" health club or anonymous track where we are not recognized or bothered. Following a really big binge, we have been known to walk stadium stairs or run back streets all night long. Above all, we want to avoid lectures, judgments or sightseeing tours as we morph from the Pillsbury Dough girls into Bionic Women. It's a tough call.

We often looked for dark hiding places to exercise, like a guilty junkie looking for a place to "shoot." We did not even have to worry about weirdoes because we can outrun them—the best of 'em. (And we start looking pretty scary ourselves after working out for six hours straight!)

Once a gentleman stopped me in the middle of my exercise-athon and handed me his business card. As he walked away, I thought he was hitting on me—how rude! But on his card he had written, "Call me for your own good" right under the printed word: Psychiatrist.

Another time, I produced the cream of the crop excuse while we were traveling on the West Coast, and all the local gyms were closed. It was pouring rain at midnight, and I had been running for hours in a six-level parking garage when Inspector Clousseau, the intrepid midnight security guard, caught me.

As soon as I stopped running, my muscles began cramping and I groaned and bowed my head, gasping for air. The security guard looked concerned and questioned me. "I am doing physical therapy that my doctors have prescribed for this condition. I have to detoxify a poison in my system, and if I stop moving, my muscles lock, and the poison eats into my body, and I can die!" The guard nervously urged me to keep going as he walked away.

"When will they find the cure?" the poor guy yelled from the other side of the garage. He actually wanted to escort me to the hospital! What excuse would I possibly give him the next night? He could not be that gullible—or could he?

Scary diet story 6

In our early twenties, we were not famous as much as infamous, and the tabloids were absolutely fascinated. We were frequently recognized, and nothing was more embarrassing than being at Denny's, chowing down after doing a TV interview. Once, a waitress and other diners asked us to autograph the menu from which we had just ordered nearly everything.

We once arrived at Los Angeles Airport after a six-hour chocolate chip cookie extravaganza on the MGM plane. We were coming off a shoot and were eating everything in sight, including unlimited cookies, candy and milk. The effects of a sugar high like this, in extreme cases, resembles taking speed. From the combination of being dehydrated from flying, bloated from bingeing, and then eating a steady stream of sweets for six hours, we could not put on our shoes, zip up our jeans or get the crumbs out of our hair fast enough.

As we landed, airport security warned us that there was a crew of paparazzi waiting for Brooke Shields and two other stars also on board the plane. We panicked—we did not want the cameras to catch us—but a guardian angel security guard came to our rescue. While Brooke and the other celebrities were picked up by their humble rides, we were chagrined to realize that a stretch limo was waiting for us—and attracting a lot of unwanted attention. Naturally, the growing media crowd figured form the size of our ride that Liz Taylor or Madonna were hidden inside. Not!

Finally, the limo driver pulled up to a rear exit, but a few photographers followed him. Suddenly, it seemed like there were searchlights beaming down at us from a helicopter—all of those fat-searching camera lights were terrifying. We made a run for it, with the help of our guardian angel, and I dove headfirst through the driver's seat window—not a pretty picture. Shane grabbed an MGM umbrella, hid behind it, and ran into the limo. In the tabloids the next day, my sister was misidentified in People magazine as a certain well-known actress—who must have been pretty upset. But we were saved again.

Chapter 4

Menus, recipes, charts and a nutritional survey

Here we offer you sensible sample menus of different types of diets that worked for us in recovery. As you may realize by now, no single eating plan satisfies everybody, but we offer these strategies with the hope that you'll find a healthy, dietary fit. Remember: You won't lose and keep weight off permanently if you don't eat enough calories. Be sensible, exercise regularly and drink lots of water throughout the day:

Exercise buffs (or maintenance plan)

If you're exercising moderately, you need to keep fueling up throughout the day to sustain stamina for both exercise and the rigors of daily life. This nutritious program is also beneficial for dieters who are close to goal weight and want to maintain their figure.

Breakfast
1-2 cups 10-grain cereal or slow-cooking oatmeal, 1 medium fruit
1 cup of milk and/or orange juice
Snack
1 cup of nonfat yogurt (sprinkled 2 oz. seeds, nuts or raisins)
Lunch
Two slices rye bread or 5-7 crackers with 3 oz. nonfat cream cheese
1 cup of lentil soup, or 1 can of tuna, sprouts, tomato on rye
8 oz. fruit smoothie
Snack:
1 cup of lowfat cottage cheese or glass of milk
Dinner
3-4 oz. chicken, 1 cup black-eyed beans, 1 cup baked yams, 1 slice sprouted wheat bread; or 3 oz. tofu and 2 cups steamed vegetables mixed with 1 cup noodles or rice, and served with a small fruit salad

Slow metabolism—need to lose weight"

Breakfast
2 egg whites and 1 yolk mixed in an herb omelet

On the side (or inside omelet), mix 1/2 cup sliced peach or pear with 1 cup nonfat yogurt and cinnamon
Snack
1 hard-boiled egg and 1 cup baby carrots
Lunch
3-4 oz. meat or fish, beans or lentils; and 1 large fruit
Snack
1 cup lowfat yogurt or nonfat cottage cheese
Dinner
3-4 oz. meat or fish, and 2 cups salad: mix raw greens with nonfat yogurt dressing or a dab of olive oil with vinegar

High-protein menu
Breakfast
Egg omelet (1 full egg, 2 egg whites) mixed with 3-4 oz. nonfat cream cheese
Sprinkle with cinnamon and add sliced berries
Snack
Turkey jerky or 3 oz. lean turkey on 1 slice sprouted bread with mustard
Lunch
3-4 oz. tofu mixed with 1 cup steamed cauliflower, squash and mushrooms
Sprinkle nonfat cheese on top and melt
Snack
1/2 cup lowfat cottage cheese and 1 thick slice of avocado (or handful of nuts)
Dinner
3-4 oz. grilled fish or meat and 1 cup slow-cooking beans
Gelatin desert (no carbs)

High-carb menu
Breakfast
1 cup slow-cooking oatmeal or 10-grain cereal, 1/2 melon or 1 cup sliced fruit
Snack
1 cup air-popped popcorn or 1 cereal bar
Lunch
A steamed yam or potato, 1 cup steamed peas with garlic or split pea soup, 1 cup sliced carrots or other colorful veggies
Snack
4-5 rye crackers dipped in nonfat yogurt mixed with salsa
Dinner
1 cup cooked brown basmati rice mixed with 1 cup black-eyed peas and lentils; 1 cup cut-raw vegetables; and 1 whole-wheat pita. One cup fresh fruit salad

All-you-can-eat diet

Plan to eat three meals and two fuel-rich (carb) snacks per day, but choose one meal and allow yourself to eat whatever you want for that hour. During that time, since you're eating a lot anyway, try not to mix proteins and carbohydrates. This has worked for us because that one magic meal is exciting and satiating. It also works because we don't go hog-wild (pun intended). In other words, the allowable foods in that hour are not cookies, prime rib or hunks of cheese!

Breakfast
1 cup puffed cereal with skim milk, topped with 1/2 cup berries
Snack
Bran muffin or bagel with 1 Tbs. sugarless jam
Lunch
A handful of olives), 3 oz. lowfat cheese, 3 oz. sliced cold cuts, one large pickle
Snack
1/2 cup dried fruit mix or one cup orange juice
Dinner
Protein and fats only; eat slowly and thoroughly. Start with one cup of chicken broth; then eat very lean portions of skinless poultry or steak, unlimited crawfish or shellfish with cocktail sauce and lemon; try 1 cup of beans cooked how you like them. Eat as many steamed veggies as you want with your meal—prepare without butter or oils.

Fuel for sports—carbohydrate loading

Four or more days of:

Breakfast
3-4 egg whites in omelet filled with 3 oz. ricotta cheese or nonfat cream cheese; herbal tea with lemon
Lunch
1 cup mixed beans (lentils, pintos, black-eyed peas, kidney beans, soybeans) mixed with handful scallions and steamed Brussels sprouts (spice to taste); 3-4 oz. grilled chicken or turkey breast
Dinner
3-4 oz. grilled fish steamed, grilled or roasted with 1 cup sliced, raw veggies with balsamic vinegar and spices
Dessert
Blend 4 oz. nonfat milk, 4 oz. nonfat yogurt, 1 lemon (peel also), 2 oz. seeds and/or nuts, cinnamon, and a few drops vanilla extract

Cleansing diet samples
(supervised fasting for 1-3 days)

Choose one:
8 oz. fresh grapefruit, lemon, lime juice—3 hours apart
8 oz. celery, bell pepper, cucumber—3 hours apart
8 oz. fresh apple juice with spirulina—3 hours apart
1 oz. wheat grass juice—2 hours apart

Food combining menu

We know this is controversial—and outdated in most nutrition circles—but we feel the separation of nutrients simplifies the digestion process, and it also tastes really good. (All of these menus are nutrient-dense and balanced.)

Breakfast
2 cups mixed fruit, all fruit must be eaten without other carbs or proteins, do not eat melon with other fruit

Lunch
2 cups any complex carbs (starch), including wheat or rye bread, brown rice or pasta
Toss with 1-2 cups steamed vegetables only—lemon and herbs or balsamic vinegar
Do not eat fruit or protein at this meal

Dinner
4 oz. steamed or wok tofu, meat or fish, with 1-2 cups roasted or steamed vegetables only
Stir-fry lightly with soy sauce and sesame oil
No fruit or starches

Mother-to-be sample diet

The aim is to keep mom healthy, satisfied and full of energy as she experiences the myriad surprises erupting in her changing body. She will eat six small nutritious meals spaced out every two hours. Drink lots of water, skim milk and fresh juice all day long.

Meal 1
1 cup granola, kashi or muesli with 1 cup skim milk and 1 medium fruit (or 1/2 cup raisins tossed with fresh-squeezed juice)

Meal 2
1 cooked egg, 1 piece dry rye toast, warm water with lemon

Meal 1
1 cup nonfat yogurt with 2 oz. raw seeds and nuts and 1 Tbs. bran

Meal 4
Half a pita filled with avocado slices, 1/8 cup nonfat sour cream, 3 oz. tuna

with onions or scallions, tomatoes, celery and cucumber
Meal 5
1 cup lentil or vegetable soup; 1 cup chopped raw carrots, celery or green veggies.
Meal 5
3 oz. grilled salmon (or other fish high in essential fatty acids, such as halibut or bluefish), a baked yam or potato. Mix 1-2 cups fresh greens with olive oil, organic apple cider vinegar or fruit salad

Post-pregnancy sample diet

You're bound to be exhausted and a little frustrated after the baby arrives. Enlist support from your mate and loved ones to eat filling, stamina-sustaining meals throughout the day. Eat most of your carbs in the AM to fuel up first thing in the morning, drink milk and juices to keep blood sugar steady, and pump up your metabolism in the PM by eating a protein-rich dinner. Some of our post-pregnancy meals should feel like rewards for a job well done!

Breakfast
French toast (mix one full egg and two egg whites with 1-2 oz. skim milk as batter)
Dip two pieces 10-grain bread in batter, fry in pan lightly sprayed with olive oil
Garnish with cinnamon and berries
Drink herb tea or decaf coffee and 1 cup skim milk
Snack
1/2 cup nonfat cottage cheese with either 1 cup chopped veggies or sliced fruit
Lunch
3-4 oz. grilled tofu or fish tossed with 1-2 cups steamed broccoli, cauliflower, bell peppers and tomatoes
Top with melted cheese sauce made from 2 oz. nonfat cheese, 3 Tbs. skim milk, diced garlic, scallions and minced parsley
Bake at 350° F until casserole becomes browned on top
Drink tall glass of mineral water with lime
Snack
3 oz. string cheese or turkey jerky and 1 sliced apple
Dinner
2 cups slivered raw green vegetables and 2 shredded carrots
Dressing: 1/2 cup nonfat yogurt or sour cream with 1 cup diced red onion, tomatoes, garlic, and olives
Mix with 3-4 oz. roasted turkey or chicken breast
Drink sparkling water mixed with 1 Tbs. apple juice or heat 1 cup apple cider

Our favorite recipes

BAKED APPLE DELIGHT (one per serving)

Core a large apple, but leave the bottom on the apple so nothing leaks out. Spray olive oil on the surface. Place raisins, berries and chopped almonds in a lightly oiled fry pan and grill. Mix with 1/2 cup of cooked oatmeal and 1/2 tsp. of cinnamon. Place mixture in the core of the apple and bake at 350° F until soft (10-15 minutes).

LAYERED YOGURT CUP (serves two)

Mix two cups of chopped berries, peaches, bananas, apples, oranges, or fruit and season with 1/2 cup chopped mixed nuts (peanuts, almonds or pecans). Toss mixture into one cup of non-fact yogurt and add:
1 Tbs. lecithin
1 Tbs. protein powder
1 tsp. cinnamon and nutmeg
1/2 tsp. vanilla extract
Layer in a large, fancy, tall wine or champagne glass: Fruit first, then a thin sprinkle of nuts. Repeat until you have a colorful, layered glass with nuts on top. Chill in freezer until semi-frozen.

FRUIT CHEESE BLINTZ (serves one)

1/2 cup mixed fruit
1 oz. lowfat cream cheese
Mix a batter of:
1 egg, 2 egg whites
2 Tbs. soy powder
2 Tbs. wheat bran
2 Tbs. skim milk
1/2 tsp. cinnamon
Put batter in pan sprayed with olive oil. Layer 1 oz. nonfat cream cheese and simmer until cheese melts. Place thin layer of chopped blueberries or soft fruit on top and roll thin, (crepe-like) omelet with fruit and cheese on top. Roll from one end to the other.

PROTEIN FRUIT SMOOTHIE (serves one)

Blend: 1/2 cup soy milk
1/2 cup nonfat yogurt
1 Tbs. brewer's yeast
1/2 banana
1 tangerine
1/2 apple
4 ice cubes

FRUIT FRENCH TOAST (serves one)

Make a batter from:

1 egg, 2 egg whites
1 Tbs. cinnamon
1 Tbs. nutmeg
1 Tbs. protein powder
6 Tbs. skim or soy milk
Spray frying pan with olive oil and lightly grill 1/2 cup berries, apples and/or peaches, mixed. Set aside. Put slices of 10-grain bread in batter, grill and top with warm fruit topping.

VEGGIE CHEESE OMELET (serves one)
1 egg, 2 egg whites (or egg beaters)
1-2 oz. nonfat cheddar cheese
1/4 cup chopped tomato, parsley, scallions, condiments and your choice of hot sauce
1/4 cup of lightly grilled mushrooms, onions and bell peppers
Spray pan with olive oil. Pour in egg batter and layer with chopped vegetables and grilled vegetables. Sprinkle cheese and fold over when solid, but not yet finished. Let sit until fully cooked.

OAT-APPLE-CARROT MUFFIN (makes 8-10 muffins)
3 Tbs. soy protein powder
2 oz. oat bran
2 oz. whole wheat flour
1/2 cup nonfat milk
1/2 Tbs. canola oil
1 egg , 1 egg white
1/2 cup shredded carrots and apples
Blend ingredients, fill muffin cups sprayed with olive oil. Bake at 325° F for about 45 minutes.

BEAN SOUP (serves four)
3 cups black-eyed peas
1/2 cup lentils
1/2 cup split peas
1/2 cup cooked pinto beans
1/2 kidney beans
Soak for four hours and simmer two hours over low heat. Turn off heat and mix three cups chopped broccoli, mushrooms, celery, bell pepper and onions. Season to taste. Replace lid and let the dish sit for one hour.

VEGETABLE QUICHE (serves two)
2 full eggs
4 egg whites
4 oz. shredded lowfat cheese
2 cups vegetables cut into thin strips: tomatoes, mushrooms, broccoli, cauli-

flower, red peppers. Steam with peas.
Place vegetables in pan, pour egg batter on top. Spread shredded cheese on top,
sprinkle with garlic, salt and pepper. Bake at 325 F for 15-20 minutes.

EGGPLANT LASAGNA (serves 4)
1 large eggplant
2 large beefsteak tomatoes
10 mushrooms
6 oz. nonfat ricotta
8 oz. nonfat mozzarella
1/2 cup minced parsley, garlic and black olives mixed with 2 tsp. oregano
Slice eggplant into thin strips and grill lightly with tomato and mushroom
slices. Layer in small casserole pan (sprayed with olive oil) in this order:
Eggplant on bottom,
Layer of ricotta,
Layer of minced parsley, garlic and olives.
Shred mozzarella cheese.
Spread tomato and mushroom slices.
Sprinkle a bit parmesan cheese on top and bake for 1 hour at 350° F or until
top is melty.

VEGETABLE OR TOFU BURGER (serves one)
1 tofu patty
1/2 oz. shredded nonfat cheese
2 slices each: tomato, cucumber and mushroom
2 leaves green lettuce
Heat whole grain bread (100 percent rye is best) and spread with nonfat
yogurt, mustard and dill.

TEMPE STIR FRY (serves 2)
6-8 oz. seaweed tempe
2 cups chopped vegetables (cauliflower, celery, snow peas, onions or scallions,
bell pepper, mushrooms, etc.)
Spray olive oil in stir fry pan and slowly add low-sodium soy sauce. Stir until
vegetables are slightly cooked, adding 1 Tbs. peanut or sesame oil, if needed.

SHRIMP OR CRAWFISH DIP (serves 2)
4-6 oz. crawfish (or shrimp)
4-6 oz. lowfat cottage cheese
3 cups chopped scallions, onions, parsley, cucumbers and celery
1 Tbs. lemon or lime juice
1/2 tsp. garlic salt and pepper
Mix together and serve on Rye Crisp crackers or heated mini-pita pieces or
baked no-oil, no-salt health chips.

CHICKEN PASTA SALAD (serves one)
3 oz. chopped, grilled chicken breast
1/3 cup spinach noodles, steamed with 1/2 Tbs. olive oil.
1 cup chopped vegetables (cabbage, red onion, celery, cucumber, carrot, tomatoes, artichoke hearts, etc.)
Toss, hot or cold, with dressing mixed to taste: organic apple cider, vinegar and lemon juice mixed with olive oil. Mix herbs and condiments, chives and garlic.

PITA BREAD FILLER (serves one)
1 whole wheat pita bread, heated slightly
1/2 cup nonfat ricotta cheese
1/2 cup avocado
1/2 cup chopped cucumber, tomatoes, celery, and onions
Mash avocado with lemon, white pepper and garlic salt. Mix with vegetables and ricotta. Place in pita with handful of sprouts.

SALMON ALMOND DINNER (serves one)
3-4 oz. salmon, thinly sliced
1/2 cup sliced almonds
1 cup chopped mushrooms, parsley, yellow onion, and red peppers
batter from 2 egg whites
1/2 cup salsa as optional seasoning
Put fish in batter, then cover with chopped almonds. Spray olive oil on a piece of foil or a broiling pan, place fish on sprayed pan. Cover fish with chopped vegetables and sprinkle parmesan cheese on top. Heat in broiler until done, 7-10 minutes; add salsa. Sprinkle with lemon juice and garnish.

STUFFED PEPPERS (serves one)
Core bell pepper and fill with 1/2 cup steamed vegetables (cauliflower, broccoli, mushrooms, and onions)
1/2 cup mix cooked beans
1/2 cup basmati rice
Put slice of tomato on top and sprinkle with parmesan cheese. Spray olive oil on outside pepper shells. Bake at 350 F until shell is soft and top is brown.

MEXICAN LAYER CASSEROLE (serves one)
Prepare sauce:
1/2 cup nonfat sour cream
1/2 cup avocado
1/4 cup minced tomato, garlic, parsley and scallions
Lightly grill:
3-4 oz. chicken, tofu or tempe, spray with olive oil, and top with 1/4 cup red onions, celery and mushrooms.
Heat a whole wheat tortilla and spray lightly with olive oil. Place tortilla on bottom of casserole pan. Put protein and vegetable mix on tortilla. Layer with 2

oz. nonfat shredded cheese. Bake at 325 F for 15 minutes. Top with 1 Tbs. salsa, and sprinkle with sliced olives.

Food groups and exchanges

These represent approximate amounts in our menus and diet plans and can be interchanged within the same food group. Feel free to experiment and discover the recipes, which serve you best.

Fats and oils

One serving: one tsp. butter, margarine or 1Tbs. salad dressing or mayonnaise; or 2 oz. seeds and nuts or 1/5 avocado.

High-protein food items—meat and dairy substitutes

One serving is 3 oz. meat, poultry, fish; 4 oz. tofu; 3-4 Tbs. peanut butter; 1 cup cooked lentils or beans; 3 oz. sliced deli meats.

Fish and poultry

One serving is approximately 3-4 oz. fish, skinless chicken, white meat turkey or almost one can tuna; or one cup of shrimp, oysters, crab or crawfish.

Dairy

One serving is approximately one cup skim or soy milk or yogurt; one cup buttermilk, cottage cheese; 2 oz. processed cheese; 1/2 cup evaporated milk.

Grains, breads and cereals

One serving is approximately 1/2 cup cooked grains such as brown rice, pasta, millet, barley, corn, oats, dry cereals or one slice bread, pita, tortilla; or 3-5 crackers (depending on the size); or two rice cakes.

Vegetables

One serving is approximately 1/2 cup raw or cooked vegetables and beans; 1 potato. NOTE: For snacks, eat all you want of raw celery, cucumbers, endive, sea vegetables, watercress, radishes, green onions, chives, cabbage, alfalfa sprouts, bell peppers and mushrooms.

Fruit

One serving is approximately one medium-sized fruit 3/4 cup juice; 1/4 cup dried fruit; 1/2 melon; or 1/2 cup berries, cherries or grapes.

Nutritional survey

As we prepared this book, we surveyed 100 people about their diet needs and nutrition goals. Eighty percent of our anonymous respondents were women 16-45 years old. Understandably, when we asked the questions, many men didn't notice or pay as much attention as the weight-conscious women in our survey. We think you'll be as interested in their answers as we are. The first answer listed was the most popular, and the second answer warranted a lot of responses:

1. *What's the most popular diet?*
   - *Zone or protein diets*
   - *No fat, all-you-can-eat diets*

2. *What diet do you think works best?*
   - *Protein diets and organized eating programs (OA, Weight Watcher's, etc.)*
   - *Give up on diets, exercise and eat small, sensible meals.*

3. *Which diet lasts the longest?*
   - *Moderate food plans in which you lose 1-2 pounds per week.*
   - *Any diet that incorporates exercise as a "way of life."*

4. *What do you consider a perfect body—is there such a thing?*
   - *Tall and lean with great muscle tone and a speedy metabolism. "Someone who can eat anything."*
   - *Different strokes for different folks. Physical variety is the spice of life.*

5. *How long does the average diet last?*
   - *Monday through Thursday.*
   - *Until the realization hits that results are not immediate.*

6. *If diets are the number-one obsession for many people, why is there such a multitude of conflicting theories?*
   - *Because people want to believe only what they want*
   - *It is easier to buy a new fad than to do all the hard work*

7. *Is it lack of willpower, genetic predisposition, or chemical imbalance that makes a person fat?*
   - *Combination of all of the above*
   - *Combination of all of the above, plus low self-esteem*

8. *Does financial status have anything to do with eating disorders?*
   - *Most people believe it's easier to be fit if you can afford personal trainers, spa trips, personal chefs, etc.*
   - *The pressure to be "model-thin" mostly affects wealthy or high profile women.*

9. *What is the most popular "fix" besides dieting?*
   - *Plastic surgery*
   - *Falling in love*

10. *What is your main reason for wanting to diet?*
   - To look fashionably lean and to look attractive for a lover, husband or potential suitor.
   - Health reasons—to prevent heart disease, obesity, diabetes, and high blood pressure.
11. *Would you rather be rich or thin?*
   - Thin!
   - Rich, so I can afford the trainer, fat farms and fad diets!

12. *Would a dramatic weight increase in your lover be a reason to leave him or her?*
   - Women: 85% said "no way"
   - Men: 80% said "possibly"

13. *How do you view extremely obese people?*
   - They do not respect themselves.
   - They have issues which are deeper than just food consumption

14. *What is the hardest food to give up in a diet?*
   - Chocolate
   - Pizza and fast food

Scary diet story 7

In the early years, when we were feeling too fat to model, our solution was to crash-diet in the weeks leading up to the shoot or media event, and then eat afterwards—eat a lot. This punishment/reward system became a safe ritual until the will power to starve and our diet shortcuts stopped working.

After the starving phase always accompanied by over-exercising, (which lasted a few years) our subsequent bulimia practice consisted mostly of over-exercising and laxative abuse. We were not overly successful in the puke department for the first year or so of our bulimia. Then we learned this new diet secret from top models in Europe while we were on location in Paris.

We remember how graceful they looked, those international model-icons upchucking over the European toilets. Those posers were quick, efficient and utterly silent—it was a high art form. We were completely envious.

My sister Shane cannot sing, dance or act; nonetheless, I was envious of her because my sister can puke like a champ. Shane can vomit on command with one dainty, agile finger. She even tried to teach me, which must have resembled a Broadway choreographer teacher, a novice dancer and a snappy musical number called "All That Spew." At first, I thought my fingers were not long enough because I could not induce vomiting. It did not work. Then I stuck a toothbrush down my throat to help me gag. (You will be happy to know that we had impeccable hygiene and always separated our barfing toothbrushes from the regular variety.) When the toothbrushes stopped working, I even considered using the end of the toilet bowl brush. That consideration alone made me heave, but only once!

Practice makes perfect, right? I tried developing Shane's vomit-style and—nothing! Nothing but drool, a sore throat, swollen eyes, a runny nose and painful stomach rebellions.

I realized that my food disorder was utterly out of control when a good friend was horribly sick with the flu. He had been in bed for a week, and I called to check his condition. He was at his worst when he picked up the phone because, as he was telling me how much better he felt, the poor guy vomited. I was dead silent on the other end of the phone as he retched and retched. Afterwards, he came back on the line, apologizing. He said, "I'm sorry, Sia; I am so embarrassed." After I was quiet for a while, he asked if I was upset with him. "No, I'm not upset. Just jealous."

Scary diet story 8

Modeling in Paris, Milan and other European cities gave us a reputation and an attitude. While we were still in our starving stages (binges and purges were a full year or two away), we obviously did not want people to recognize our food problems or discover our all-night aerobics sessions. The most annoying part of those years was witnessing rail-thin models eat whatever they wanted, whenever they wanted, and use walks to McDonalds' as their own form of exercise.

For almost six months straight, we had the same meal everyday for lunch and dinner: a single boiled egg. We remember how they brought our meals at one five star hotel in France. The egg was placed elegantly on an expensive silver platter and served with fancy utensils. The ritual actually made the egg look very important, but extremely lonely.

Anyway, this insane diet took a toll on Shane. Let's put it delicately: she never had the opportunity to use those fancy bidet toilets. One night, she was so painfully constipated that she screamed at the top of her lungs. We finally found a hospital and my melodramatic sister was given a prescription for super-efficient laxatives. Although, we did not know it that fateful night, a new diet door opened, in more ways than one.

Free radicals and antioxidants

Free radicals are produced when cells are exposed to high oxygen concentrations that destroy cell membranes. Highly active, free radicals are present in the environment via air pollution, tobacco smoke, pesticides, hydrocarbons, rancid foods and other sources. After years of free radical exposure, constant deterioration of our cell membranes can cause degenerative diseases, such as heart disease, arthritis, cancer, hardening of the arteries, mental disorders and immune depletion. Damage to connective tissue can also promote wrinkles, loss of skin tone and increased effects of aging.

Antioxidants protect us by battling the effects of free radicals. All antioxidants, such as vitamin C, vitamin E, beta-carotene and the mineral selenium are found in foods we eat, especially in raw fruit and vegetables. Below is a brief list of some of the most important vitamins and potential antioxidants:

Vitamin A
Benefits: Builds optical system, and resists infections. Aids healthy skin and hair, strong bones and teeth. Important nutrient when pregnant.

Found in: Milk, cheese, leafy green vegetables, yams, sweet potatos, liver, egg, dairy, fish oils, fruit, melons.

Depletion symptoms: Dry eyes, night blindness, dry, itchy skin, weak tooth enamel, chronic diarrhea, bladder infections. Laxative abuse depletes vitamin A.

Beta carotene
Benefits: This antioxidant is a precursor to vitamin A. It battles infection, strengthens immune system, fights pollutants and allergies.

Found in: Green leafy vegetables, green peppers, carrots, cantaloupes, kale, peaches, mangos, nectarines, papayas, prunes, squash, sweet potato,s spinach, and sea vegetables.

Depletion symptoms: Blurred vision, kidney stones, impaired growth.

Vitamin B1
Benefits: Strengthens nervous system, immune function and increases mental capacity. Aids growth and helps stop motion sickness. Pregnancy, lactation, diuretics and oral contraceptives require increased intake. Smoking, pollutants, stress and alcohol deplete B1.

Found in: Whole grains, asparagus, brewer's yeast, nuts and seeds, wheat germ, oatmeal, red meat, dairy products.

Depletion symptoms: Edema, loss of appetite, depression, fatigue, loss of energy, poor mental abilities, insomnia, weight loss, constipation.

Vitamin B2
Benefits: Boosts energy and metabolism, promotes healthy skin and

eyes. Reduces the impact of drug toxicity and environmental chemicals. Controls cataract build-up. Extra B2 needed during pregnancy; oral contraceptive consumption, lactation, depression, use of diuretics and stress overload the demand for B2.

Found in: Milk, nuts, brewer's yeast, egg, mushrooms, yogurt, liver, kidney, cheese, whole grains.

Depletion symptoms: Skin problems, hypersensitivity to light, reddening of the cornea.

Vitamin B3

Benefits: Increases energy metabolism, helps metabolize cholesterol and sugars, enhances digestion and production of sex hormones. Good for healthy skin and nerves. May help fight acne, diarrhea and migraine headaches.

Found in: Milk, poultry, almond, avocado, brewer's yeast, fish, liver, beans, legumes, banana, whole grains, green vegetables.

Depletion symptoms: Headaches, gum disease, loss of concentration, depression, fatigue, irritability, loss of appetite, insomnia, heartburn, nausea.

Vitamin B5

Benefits: An antioxidant important for immune system function and adrenal activity. May help prevent arthritis and lower cholesterol. Helps fight infection, strengthen antibodies; decrease stress, fatigue and nerve disorders. Enhances healing after surgery.

Found in: Brewer's yeast, brown rice, poultry, yams, whole grains, liver, kidney, broccoli, legumes, peas, bran, molasses.

Depletion symptoms: Insomnia, vomiting, lack of energy and coordination. May cause skin problems, dizzy spells, digestive malfunctions and foot pain.

Vitamin B6

Benefits: Helps metabolize fat and protein and helps make red blood cells. Eases nausea and skin disorders.

Found in: Meat, fish, fruit, wheat germ, egg yolk, cantaloupes, cabbage, milk, brewer's yeast.

Depletion symptoms: Anemia, nervous system disorders, insomnia, skin abnormalities and loss of muscle function.

Vitamin B12

Benefits: Boosts production of healthy red blood cells, hinders anemia, enhances children's growth.

Found in: Meat, shellfish, eggs, dairy products.

Depletion symptoms: Anemia, poor appetite, growth retardation, loss of energy, pale skin.

Biotin (member of B complex)
Benefits: Aids energy metabolism, speeds up growth and boosts metabolic function.
Found in: Brewer's yeast, most fruits and vegetables
Depletion symptoms: Appetite fluctuations, energy loss, decreased muscle function.

Choline (B complex) and Inositol (B complex)
Benefits: Aids liver function, metabolism and the breakdown of fat.
Found in: Egg yolk, green leafy vegetables, legumes, yeast, liver, wheat germ (choline). Fruit, nuts, whole grains, milk, meat, brewer's yeast (inositol).
Depletion symptoms: Dysfunction of the liver, problems with fat breakdown and hardening of arteries.

Folic acid (member of B complex)
Benefits: Builds new cells, helps protein metabolism and aids growth. Builds red blood cells in bone marrow.
Found in: Dark green leafy vegetables, liver, legumes, kidney, yeast.
Depletion symptoms: Anemia, heartburn, constipation, depression, frequent infections.

Vitamin C
Benefits: Maintains healthy teeth, gums and bones. Fights infection, speeds up wound healing, builds connective tissue.
Found in: Citrus fruit, broccoli, Brussels sprouts, kale, papaya, mango, cabbage, red and green peppers. Cooking destroys efficacy of vitamin C.
Depletion symptoms: Anemia, hair loss, soft gums, tooth decay, loss of appetite, bruising, muscle degeneration, bone fragility.

Vitamin D
Benefits: Stimulates kidney function, boosts healthy teeth and bones. Vital to children's growth.
Found in: Natural sunshine, fish liver oils, fat, eggs, milk, butter.
Depletion symptoms: Rickets, tooth decay, growth retardation, loss of muscle tone and energy.

Vitamin E
Benefits: This antioxidant builds the immune system and acts as an anti-coagulant (eliminates blood clots). Helps fight heart disease and stimulates kidney function.
Found in: Wheat germ, whole wheat, green leafy vegetables, vegetable oils, meat, eggs, nuts and seeds and whole grain cereal.

Depletion symptoms: Anemia, leg cramps, weakness, decreased reproductive function and muscular disorders.

Vitamin F
Benefits: Helps growth process, helps build healthy skin, hair and glands. Lowers blood cholesterol. Helps fight heart disease.
Found in: Vegetable oils, such as soybean, peanut, safflower, cottonseed and corn oil.
Depletion symptoms: Skin disorders, such as eczema.

Vitamin K
Benefits: Aids blood clotting and liver function. Helps regulate calcium.
Found in: Milk, cabbage, liver, alfalfa sprouts, green vegetables, soybean oil, egg yolk.
Depletion symptoms: Hemorrhaging.

Vitamin P
Benefits: Protects Vitamin C. Beneficial in hypertension, may help build up resistance to colds.
Found in: Peels and pulp of all citrus fruit.
Depletion symptoms: Skin spots and weak capillary walls.

PABA
Benefits: Helps growth and folic acid assimilation.
Found in: Yeast.
Depletion symptoms: Energy loss, eczema, anemia. Causes gray hair.

Rutin
Benefits: Same as Vitamin P.
Found in: Buckwheat.
Depletion symptoms: Same as Vitamin P.

Minerals

Minerals are vital in body functions, energy, growth and healing. Constituting the very few inorganic compounds in the body, minerals also serve as electrolytes enabling the neural transmission and complementing the ionic exchange. Just like vitamins, minerals essential for optimum health, can only be obtained through proper diet. For a limited amount of time, mineral supplements will help you get all the minerals your body needs; supplements are especially useful if you are sick, tired, stressed or depleted. The best mineral supplements are ionic—do not waste your money on buying minerals in a pill form—those minerals are pure crushed rocks—your body will have just as much luck assimilating them, as it would digesting stones. Some ionic mineral supplements contain all minerals and trace elements—in the same proportions as does sea water (minus salt, of course—it is worthy of note that the mineral content of sea water is the same as that of our blood). Taking a multi-mineral ionic supplement will benefit anyone, as modern-day food is often mineral-poor; however, for some people taking additional supplementation of particular minerals may be of use.

With age, mineral assimilation reduces. The body's ability to assimilate and hold minerals and sodium affects the body's ability to hold water—our cells do not appreciate distilled water; only water with a certain electrolyte balance is of use. A baby is made of 75% water. A grown man is 50-70 percent water. The older we are, the less water our cells retain, which phenomenon is one of the factors affecting both the appearance of our skin and the internal health of our bodies. Below is a brief list of some of the most important, minerals:

Boron   Boron helps build healthy bones and muscle. Boron is only needed in trace amounts. The elderly benefit from boron supplements because it helps absorb calcium. Sources—leafy greens, apples, carrots, nuts and grains.

Calcium   Calcium is the most abundant mineral in the body, yet it seems to be the most deficient, especially in women who have "female problems." Calcium has to be in a proper proportion with sodium, potassium and magnesium to make our bodies work like a clock—from relaxing muscles to regulating our heartbeat. Calcium absorption is tricky; it also depends on vitamin D consumption. Calcium is most important for healthy bones and teeth, but it can also be useful in lowering cholesterol. Calcium deficiency can lead to brittle, aching joints, eczema, high cholesterol, heart palpitations, high blood pressure, insomnia, muscle cramps, numbness and dental problems (especially important for athletes). Oxalic acid found in Kale (also high in calcium), spinach, beet, greens, and cocoa make calcium hard to absorb. Phytic acid (bran layer of grains) mixed with dairy also make calcium hard to absorb. Calcium shots are given to rehab patients to relax. Sources—dairy, salmon, clams, broccoli, greens, Kale, almonds, brewer's yeast, oats, soy product, bancha tea and molasses.

Note: Some researchers believe that calcium molecules in dairy and meat are too big to break down.

Chromium   Chromium is needed for energy because it is involved in the metabolism of glucose. It also helps synthesize cholesterol, fat and protein, and helps stabilize blood sugar in hypoglycemics and diabetics. Deficiency can lead to anxiety, fatigue, glucose intolerance and arterial diseases. Sources—brewer's yeast, brown rice, cheese, meat and whole grains.

Copper   Copper aids zinc and vitamin C; helps energy, healing, hair and skin coloring and the formation of bones and red blood cells. Deficiency can lead to osteoporosis, skin problems, anemia, boldness, weakness and respiratory dysfunction. Sources—almonds, avocados, garlic, liver, mushrooms, seafood and green leafy vegetables.

Germanium   Germanium detoxifies, blocks free radicals and increases cell strength. Helps cells neutralize and delete of toxins. Stimulates interferon.

Iodine   This mineral is needed only in trace amounts. Iodine helps metabolize fat and maintain thyroid health. Deficiency can lead to a mental retardation, breast cancer, fatigue or weight gain. Sources—salt, seafood, Kelp, dulse and garlic.

Iron   Iron is the most important factor in the production of hemoglobin. It is vital for a healthy immune system and energy. Excess iron, however, can cause problems and even lead to diseases. Deficiency symptoms include anemia, bone and hair problems, fatigue, nervousness, obesity and slow mental reactions. Sources—eggs, fish, liver, meat, poultry, leafy greens, whole grains, almonds, blackstrap, molasses and dried fruit.

Magnesium   Magnesium assists calcium and potassium in their functions. It is also important for enzyme activity, the body's pH balance and helps with depression and PMS. Deficiency can lead to insomnia, confusion, poor digestion and even diabetes; severe deficiency can cause cardiac arrest, asthma and depression. Magnesium/calcium ratio should be ½. Sources—dairy, fish, meat, seafood, apples, avocados, bananas, garlic, kelp, nuts and whole grains.

Manganese   Manganese is important for anemics. It controls fat metabolism and blood sugar levels; contributes to a healthy immune system. Deficiency symptoms include confusion, eye and hearing problems, memory loss, tremors and can even lead to high cholesterol, convulsions and breast ailments. Sources—avocados, nuts, seaweed, whole grains, egg yolks and parsley.

Molybdenum   Only small amounts are needed for cell function. Helps with gum disorders. Deficiency can cause cancer and make older men impotent. Sources—beans, grains and green leafy vegetables.

Phosphorus   Phosphorus is needed for bone and tooth formation, cell growth, heart and kidney function. Phosphorus should be balanced with magnesium and calcium. Deficiencies, though rare, can lead to anxiety, bone pain, weakness, numbness and weight problems. Sources—asparagus, bran, corn, brewer's yeast, dairy, eggs, fish, dried fruit, nuts, seeds, salmon and whole grains.

Potassium   This mineral is vital for the nervous system and heart rhythm and can prevent strokes, muscle problems and water retention. The elderly are often depleted of potassium, which depletion can cause weakness and circulation problems. Deficiency symptoms include skin problems, confusion, constipation, depression, diarrhea, reflex problems, heart and growth impairment, high cholesterol, insomnia, muscle fatigue, nausea, respiratory distress and salt retention. Potassium, like sodium, is an electrolyte (a dissolved salt which plays an important part in the body's fluid balance and brain chemistry stabilization). Potassium deficiency can also cause depression, acne, constipation, bloating, weakness, high cholesterol, reflex impairment, nausea and respiratory distress. Sources—dairy, fish, legumes, whole grains, chicken, bananas, apricots, dried fruit, peanuts, potatoes and leafy greens.

Selenium   Selenium, like iron, zinc, iodine and fluoride, is a trace mineral. Only small amounts are needed for important functions such as boosting the immune system and slowing down the aging process. Selenium is also an antioxidant, like vitamins C and E, preventing abnormal oxidation of body fat that can cause cancer. Deficiency can lead to cancer, heart disease, growth impairment, infections and sterility. Sources—Brazil nuts, brewer's yeast, seafood, whole grains, garlic and egg yolks.

Silicon   Silicon is necessary for the formation of bones, tissue, nails, skin and hair. Silicon helps prevent Alzheimer's disease and osteoporosis. Sources—alfalfa, beets, brown rice, soybeans, whole grains & leafy greens.

Sodium   Sodium is vital for the body's pH balance and water balance. Sodium efficiency is rare but can lead to anorexia, cramps, fatigue, depression, heart palpitations, vomiting, confusion and muscle impairment. Sources—almost all foods contain some sodium, especially pickled foods, canned foods and dairy products.

Sulfur   Sulfur is an acid forming mineral which helps resist bacteria, stimulate bile secretion, protect against toxins and slow down aging process. Deficiency causes skin problems. Sources—Brussels sprouts, eggs, garlic, dried beans, wheat germ, kale, soybeans, meat and onions.

Vanadium   Vanadium is needed in growth and reproduction. Vanadium also helps reduce cholesterol level and aids bone and teeth formation. Deficiency has been linked to cardiovascular and kidney diseases, reproductive problems and infant mortality. Vanadium is not easily absorbed. Sources—dill, fish, olives, meat, radishes and whole grains.

Zinc   Zinc is responsible for helping cells reproduce. Zinc is present in all human tissue and is essential for enzymatic activity in the body. Zinc is also vital for reproductive functions, skin care and a healthy immune system (especially helps healing wounds). Zinc also helps fight free radicals. Deficiency may result in loss of taste and smell. White spots or peeling nails can be a symptom of zinc deficiency, which can also cause acne, fatigue, growth impairment, hair loss, high cholesterol level, impotence, infections, memory loss, colds, the flu and slow wound healing.

Minerals also help maintain the blood pH at 7.35-7.45. A modern day bad diet usually causes excess acids to be dumped into the blood. If minerals are not supplied in the diet, the body will desperately rob minerals from the teeth, bones, hair, etc. (The body doesn't think those organs are essential). A clean diet of raw vegetables and fruit ensures that the body would not rob from those places. Of course, too much carbon dioxide with no acids can cause hyperventilation. Unlike vitamins, minerals should not be taken with meals.

Vitamins and minerals are ions and salts. Our body only utilizes nutrients only when it recognizes them during digestion. The body is not a slot machine. It is, therefore, important to get vitamins and minerals through a wholesome diet, or vitamins, which are food-derived, in order to make sure the body recognizes them during digestion.

Vitamins are considered fragmented foods, and may be flushed out without being absorbed. Because too much vitamin C cancels vitamin B's effects, and calcium does not work without magnesium, or with iron; it is best to let nature take care of the biochemical breakdown. A simple multivitamin is biochemically balanced.

It is said, though, that a sailor (in the old days) suffering with scurvy (lack of vitamin C), could have had orange peels applied to his skin, and his body would have assimilated that vitamin C from the orange peels. In cases of extreme deficiency, the body will utilize anything to get what it needs

Possible energy and diet aids

The term "ergogenic aids" implies a source of energy or a performance enhancer. Certain supplements, home remedies and amino acids (protein molecules that perform many different tasks in the body) have all—

at one time—been touted as supplements that aid metabolism and nutrition. Below we list some of the better-known varieties, in addition to providing a few of our own. Please note that many ergogenics are controversial and still mandate extensive testing. As always, consult a professional before taking anything.

♦*Shiitake mushrooms*	Called oyster mushrooms when fresh. Used often in Asian medicine to prevent high blood pressure and heart disease, and to reduce cholesterol.
♦*Tyrosine*	Growth hormone stimulant; builds adrenaline and thyroid hormones. Source of quick energy; may stimulate fat metabolism.
♦ *L-Glutathione*	Works with cysteine and glutamine to neutralize toxicity of chemotherapy, X-rays and other medical treatments. Reduces liver toxicity.
♦ *Egg yolk lecithin*	Powerful source of choline and phosphatides, used in treatment of immune deficiency diseases. Must be kept in a very cool area.
♦ *GLA (Gamma Linoleic Acid)*	Derived from essential fatty oils (evening primrose, black currant and borrage seed). Energy source for cells, insulation for nerve fibers.
♦ *DiMethyl-Glycine*	Once known as Vitamin B-15. Energy stimulant used by athletes for endurance and stamina. Warning: As with many ergogenics, new studies show that too much DMG can destroy normal metabolic response, and cause fatigue and depression.
♦ *Octacosanol*	Wheat germ derivative that combats fatigue and enhances oxygen utilization during exercise.

◆ *Reishi mushrooms*	Tonic to increase vitality and enhance immunity. Help eliminate side effects of chemotherapy and other medical treatments.
◆ *Wheat Germ Oil*	Rich in B vitamins, Vitamin E and iron. Keep in a very cool area.
◆ *Astragalus*	Helps immune system, creates better circulation; helps lower blood pressure.
◆ *Pycnogenol*	Bioflavonoid extract made from pine bark, grapeseed and other fruit. Highly concentrated and may prove more effective than vitamins E or C as a potential antioxidant.
◆ CoQ 10	Increases cellular energy. Found in rice bran, wheat germ, beans, nuts, fish, eggs and seeds. The body's ability to assimilate this co-enzyme lessens with age.
◆ *Methionine*	A B-complex nutrient that prevents fats from accumulating in the organs such as liver and arteries. Prevents allergies.
◆ *Cysteine*	Works with Vitamins C, E and selenium. Stimulates white cell activity in the immune system and improves iron absorption.

All about enzymes

Enzymes are protein molecules, which control and enhance chemical reactions in the body. Most enzymes act in cooperation with other enzymes and nutrients, such as vitamins and minerals, to make the body function optimally. There are thousands of enzymes in a single cell, and without enzymes we would not be able to breathe, digest food or function.

There are two groups of enzymes: metabolic enzymes which regulate metabolism, repair injuries and fight disease; and digestive enzymes which process carbohydrates, protein and fat into the body and also regulate the food we eat.

Because starch breaks down in the mouth, we shouldn't wash away saliva enzymes with liquids. It is best to eat our cereals dry. The prime reason why babies get colic is because they can swallow food without chewing it. Since baby food contains starch, complete digestion does not occur. Research has shown that by eating diverse food groups separately, we allow enzymes to complete digestion quickly and perfectly. Starch breaks down in the mouth, protein-in the stomach, fat and fruit-in the lower intestine. With perfect digestion, protein takes 4 hours; starch and fat-3 hours, and fruit-2 hours. Poor enzyme distribution may take more than a day to digest a meal. Also, excess meat eating forces the stomach to produce too much hydrochloric acid, which may also cause digestive problems.

ENZYMES	
• Amylase	Digests starches in the mouth.
• Bromelain	Aids digestion of fat. An anti-inflammatory food enzyme. You can find it in pineapple.
• Catalase Antioxidant	Helps fight free radicals.
• Cellulase	Enables cellulose digestion. Found in most vegetable fiber.
• Chymotrypsin	Helps neutralize the stomach acid when semi-digested food passes from the stomach into the small intestine.
• Diastase	Enables digestion of vegetable starch.
• Glutathion Peroxidase	An antioxidant enzyme which turns free radicals into oxygen and water.
• Lactase	Enables digestion of lactose (milk sugar). Very common.
• Lipase	Breaks down fat in the stomach.
• Mycozyme	Plant enzyme that helps digest starches.
• Pancreatin	Important for prevention of degenerative diseases. Animal pancreas derivative. Helps digestion.
• Papain and chymopapain	Derived from papaya. Helps digest protein (vegetable pepsin).
• Pepsin	Breaks down protein. Can help digest 3500 times its weight in protein.
• Protease	Digests protein.
• Rennin	Helps digest cow's milk.
• Trypsin	Breaks down fat, protein and starches. Secreted by the pancreas.

Cooking destroys enzymes. Raw foods do not require as much digestive work from the body because they provide their own enzymes to work with ours. When we do not absorb a nutrient, we may manifest a deficiency of that nutrient, and, in some cases, need enzyme supplementation to help us absorb what we need. Papayas are one of the best natural sources of enzymes. Other natural sources include sprouts, bananas and avocados.

All about herbs

Herbs can be remedies, performance boosters, energy enhancers and even deadly—if taken in irresponsible doses. For hundreds of years, as prescribed by learned alternative healers, herbs have been used to treat a huge variety of conditions, such as mild burns and indigestion, as cosmetic supplements and as cures for serious medical problems.

Alfalfa Carries large amounts of calcium, magnesium, phosphorus, chlorophyll, Vitamin C, and other vitamins and minerals.

Aloe vera Gel or cream soothes burns or small wounds. Lubricates skin and improves healing. Aloe Vera juice has been known to treat acne and balance the endocrine system. Can help prevent constipation.

Black cohosh Helps reduce edema. Eases PMS and menstrual symptoms, helps fight nerve dysfunction, reduce blood pressure and prevent headache and arthritis pain.

Capsicum Increases thermogenesis for weight loss, especially when combined with caffeine herbs or ephedra (ma huang). Increases circulation.

Cayenne cream Eliminates cramping of muscles; helps other sport injuries.

Dandelion root Purifies the skin, liver, blood and endocrine system.

Echinacea Strengthens the immune system, especially against infection.

Garlic Has an antibiotic effect; fights infection.

Ginger Decreases cramping, indigestion, nausea, coughs, sinusitis and sore throat. A warming circulatory stimulant and body-cleansing herb.

Ginkgo biloba improves memory and concentration.

Ginseng Herb for energy and rejuvenation.

Goldenseal Works as a natural antibiotic; fights colds. Natural antibiotic.

Green tea Long-used as a beneficial fasting tea. Contains antioxidants and anti-allergens.

Guarana/Kola nut   Natural stimulant like ma huang, but contains caffeine, not ephedrine.

Kava   Helps calm nervous system without side effects. Enhances sleep. Naturally enhances serotonin release.

Licorice root   Fights viruses and symptoms of herpes.

Ma huang   Natural herb that stimulates the adrenals and expands bronchial tubes, but causes constriction of blood vessels. Acts as a stimulant (contains ephedrine).

Red clover   Has alkaline effect on the body. Contains large amounts of minerals.

Rosemary   Antioxidant herb; a strong brain and memory stimulant. Effective for circulatory toning, stress, tension and depression.

Saw palmetto   Helps prostate problems.

St. john's wort   This natural form of Prozac combats herpes. Effective relaxant.

Tea tree oil   Antiseptic and antifungal agent. Helps cure athlete's foot.

Valerian root   Helps insomnia without side effects or addiction.

White willow   Analgesic, anti-inflammatory and astringent. Has aspirin-like effect on arthritis and headaches.

Yellow dock root   High content of iron to prevent energy loss. Helps circulation, reduces skin eruptions and pale coloration.

Other supplements

DHEA   Hormonal supplement derived from Mexican wild yam. A precursor of testosterone. Helps to build lean muscle tissue, burn fat and give energy. We have it in our bodies, but as we age, we lose it. DHEA is only useful for those who lack it or are short of it (which usually happens as we age.

Chromium picolinate   Mineral that helps build muscles and heal wounds, helps dieters who suffer from insulin sensitivity, (which, in turn, impairs the fat burning process). Helps balance blood sugar.

L-Carnitine   Amino acid that helps metabolize fat faster, gives energy.

DLPA   Amino acid; serotonin stimulant; helps depression, akin to Prozac. Produces a feeling of being full.

Melatonin   Synthetic hormone from pineal gland. There are claims that it rejuvenates and resets your body clock so you can sleep. (Useful for jet lag.)

Natural Phen-Phen   A natural copy of the drug combo of fenfluramin-phenteramine which helps weight loss by speeding up metabolism and stimulating serotonin production.

Citrimax   Extracted from citrus fruit in South America. There are claims that it breaks down and dissolves body fat easier.

Noni Natural fruit extract. Helps eliminate chronic fatigue, detoxes, cleanses, helps headache.

Essential fatty acids Essential means the body does not manufacture them, they must be supplied in nutrition. Essential fatty acids are found in some foods, such as salmon, seeds and oats. Also found in essential fatty acids are Borrage, Primrose Black Currant, therefore, needed to burn body fat. They also help women with hormone problems. If a woman is dealing with certain hormonal imbalances, her body will not let go of body fat as it serves as a suppository of estrogen.

Creatine Extracted from beef. A tablespoon of pure creatine equals the amount of creatine in 2-1/2 lbs. of beef. Allows the muscle cells to store more water increasing their energy, allowing heavier workouts and thus increasing muscle mass complications: bloating and cell imbalance.

Brewer's yeast Contains all B-complex vitamins and amino acids. Moderates glucose tolerance, lowers cholesterol, reduces stress, retards the aging process.

Bee pollen Nutritious tonic and full-spectrum building and rejuvenating substance.

Royal jelly Supplies key nutrients for energy, mental alertness and general well-being. Enhances immunity. Rich source of pantothenic acid which fights stress, fatigue and insomnia.

Oats Metabolic stimulant which balances body chemistry. Nerve and gland restorative.

Scary diet story 9

One night while we were struggling through recovery, an Alcoholics Anonymous (AA) meeting was held next to our Overeaters Anonymous (OA) meeting. And, as I was passing through the communal hallway, a sweet guy in AA recovery flirtatiously asked where I was going. Of course I said I was in the hip AA crowd. I had rather he envision me boozing instead of barfing! Of course, I made sure we never met in the hallway again.

Scary diet story 10

The car was the most exciting place to binge because it was so convenient and anonymous: a fast food restaurant on wheels. Police pulled us over a few times, thinking we were drunk when we were simply OD-ing on sugar. (When you consume that many calories quickly, you often experience the same sort of blackouts that an alcoholic does after a big drink.

This is an inflammation and excess secretion of oil on the surface of the skin, which clogs pores and attracts germs.

Symptoms: Inflamed blemishes, possible itching and scarring.

Causes: Gland and hormonal imbalance, diet high in fat, clogged pores, poor digestion, excess sugar, constipation, certain drugs and make-up, stress, radical climate changes.

AGING (Wrinkles and Fine Lines)

FOODS THAT HELP	SUPPLEMENTS THAT HELP	HERBS THAT HELP	ALSO HELPS
Keep food portions smaller and more frequent. Keep the intake of fat and oils low, especially that of saturated fat. Eat plenty of greens. Make most of your diet raw and whole foods. Eat kelp and other sea vegetables to help steady metabolism. Eat regular non-meat proteins and a lot of fruit. Minimize alcohol intake. Try bee pollen and drink a lot of water.	L-Phenylalanine, L-Arginine, L-Lysine, L-Methionine, L-Carnitine, Beta carotene, Potassium, Selenium, Zinc. EFA oils (flax seed), Vitamin B complex, with choline and inositol. Vitamin E, Calcium, Magnesium, Vitamin D, Amino acids, Melatonin, Copper.	Burdock root, Red cloves, Echinacea, Garlic, Ginseng, Ginkgo biloba, Horsetail, Licorice root, Milk thistle, Valerian root, Wild yam.	Exercise regularly. Lift weights to strengthen bones and muscles and to increase metabolism. Try yoga and meditation, take frequent vacations with loves ones. Take sunshine baths in the nude (use SPF). Participate in anti-stress programs. Eliminate smoking. Use natural laxatives or occasional colonics if there's chronic constipation (must be supervised). Get regular checkups.

Aging is a genetically controlled process, the speed of which is determined by diet, lifestyle, genetics and environment. Believe it or not, you can slow the aging process and help prevent disease with regular exercise and a stress-free, happy lifestyle.

Symptoms: Memory loss, poor immune function, joint stiffness, muscle tightness and soreness, dry skin, loss of energy.

Causes: While aging—to an extent—is inevitable, the following factors may affect the speed of aging: high stress levels, poor diet, lack of exercise, little rest and serenity, absence of sunshine, poor environment and lifestyle choices.

BAD BREATH AND BODY ODOR

FOODS THAT HELP	SUPPLEMENTS THAT HELP	HERBS THAT HELP	ALSO HELPS
Juice fast occasionally. Eat lots of greens and cultured foods, such as yogurt and tofu, to boost intestinal bacteria. Vinegar and lemon juice help digestion and breath. Drink 8-10 glasses of water daily to keep kidneys clear. Avoid red meats, fried foods, sugar, too much dairy and junk food.	Oat bran, Psyllium husks, Rice bran, Vitamin C, Acidophilus, Garlic caps, Zinc, Vitamin A & beta carotene, Vitamin B complex, plus extra B3 and B6.	Alfalfa, Goldenseal, Myrrh, Peppermint, Rosemary, Parsley.	Exercise to detox: long, slow sweats will help. Take a mineral salt bath. Baking soda is good for breath and body odor. Use natural toothpaste and rinse! Use tea tree oil mouthwash. Wear loose cotton clothes. Use crystal rocks from health store instead of commercial deodorants. Eat slowly for proper digestion. Brush teeth and clear coating off the tongue.

These uncomfortable conditions can usually be traced to a poor diet, uneven digestion and elimination and illness.

Symptoms: Foul smelling breath or body odor.

Causes: Poor diet with chlorophyll deficiency, uneven digestion, poor hygiene, stress, smoking, gum disease and tooth decay.

CELLULITE

One of the most controversial theories in heath and wellness regards cellulite. Some experts swear that this fat is produced, in part, by the body's poor circulation and elimination capabilities. Other researches would swear that cellulite is the same old body fat that's found all over the body, but which appearance looks different due to its location on hips, thighs and buttocks. What everybody DOES agree on is that cellulite is fat, fat and more fat. Older, looser skin and excess lipids contribute to the formation of cellulite.

FOODS THAT HELP	SUPPLEMENTS THAT HELP	HERBS THAT HELP	ALSO HELPS
Reduce dietary and body fat. Eat small, easily digestible meals. Use unsaturated oils. Avoid junk food. Avoid caffeine, carbnated drinks, and too much dairy. Eliminate saturated fats from your diet. Consume oat or wheat bran to lower cholesterol.	Enzyme supplements, EFA oils (flax seed or fish oils), Kelp, B complex, Lecithin, Oat or wheat bran.	Bilberry, Gotu kola, Kola nut, Butcher broom, Seaweed tea.	Start exercising at a young age. Massages may help circulation. Stimulate lymph glands with loofah. Regular aerobic exercise. Do not smoke.

Symptoms: These frustrating lumps and bumps affect women more often than men since we do store more body fat. The orange-peel appearance of this fat, especially on the lower body, is most often due to the weak, supporting connective tissues underneath the fat.

Causes: Genetics, sedentary lifestyle, being overweight as a child, chronic poor diet, deficient diet and faulty metabolism. Some also claim that hormonal problems, yo-yo dieting and drugs may increase cellulite.

MENSTRUAL PROBLEMS

Over 75 percent of women suffer form some form of menstrual problems, from pre-menstrual syndrome to cramping, bloating and heavy bleeding during menstruation. Many of these problems are partially caused by hormonal imbalances, and many researchers believe that symptoms can be moderated through proper nutrition and the use of exercise as stress relief.

FOODS THAT HELP	SUPPLEMENTS THAT HELP	HERBS THAT HELP	ALSO HELPS
Eat more lean proteins. Stay away from saturated fats. Consume foods rich in vitamin E, such as wheat germ. Try molasses for an energy boost during your period. A raw vegetarian diet during your menstruation may help. Avoid sugar, caffeine and junk foods. Eat more salmon, tuna and halibut for the essential fatty omega oils.	Make sure you take your multi-vitamin now: Vitamin K is an important supplement for heavy bleeders. Iodine helps the thyroid control the estrogen levels. Essential oils help balance hormones. Iron and antioxidants are important now. Brewer's yeast and calcium supplements may ease bloat and insomnia. Try B6 and zinc to combat water retention.	Dong quai and Chamomile tea for cramping. Licorice root or other herbal teas to battle edema. Black cohosh is excellent for uterine fibroids; burdock root and evening primrose oil is crucial for hormonal balance.	Exercise helps ease tension and balance hormones. Massage helps bring a natural rhythm and improves circulation. Lower salt intake to help bloat. Fiber helps constipation. Soy products are a natural source of estrogen and help boost the body; they also may help regulate hormonal imbalances.

FATIGUE

Symptoms: Sleep deprivation, bouts of mental depression, lethargy and possible disease.

Causes: Poor eating, protein deficiency, poor dietary habits, emotional stress, low thyroid, overwork, anemia, stress, allergies, diabetes, chronic fatigue syndrome, abuse of tobacco, caffeine, drugs or alcohol.

FOODS THAT HELP	SUPPLEMENTS THAT HELP	HERBS THAT HELP	ALSO HELPS
Adhere to high-energy diet of mostly complex carbhydrates, fresh fruit, vegetables, whole grains and legumes, including such protein sources (to allow for about 20 — 25% of protein content) as whole grains, legumes, soy, sea foods and poultry. Aim for little dietary fat. Drink high-protein drinks with spirulina or bee pollen granules and brewer's yeast. Consume foods, high in vitamins B and C and rich in iron.	Bee pollen, Amino acids (free form), Brewer's yeast, Iron, Multivitamins & minerals, Vitamin A, Chromium, Potassium, Selenium, Zinc, Vitamin B complex plus extra B12, B1, pantothenic acid and choline, DHEA, Calcium, Magnesium, L-Phenylalanine, Royal jelly.	Cayenne pepper, Gingko biloba, Gotu kola, Ginseng, Guarana, China gold.	Reduce alcohol and caffeine intake. Do not smoke. Regular cardio and strength exercises help circulation, ease stress and improve energy. Try regular massage. Get regular sunshine. Try acupressure and deep-breathing exercises.

HEALTHY HAIR

Healthy hair often comes from balanced dietary habits and a healthy, non-stressed lifestyle. In healthy hair—hair is made of protein layers called keratin—the cell walls of the hair cuticle lie flat like shingles, leaving hair soft and shiny. In damaged or overly dry hair, the cuticle shingles are broken, making hair porous and dull.

Symptoms: Excessively dry or excessively oily hair, falling hair, flaky scalp, split ends, lack of bounce and elasticity.

Causes: Poor diet, lack of protein, recent illness and drug use.

FOODS THAT HELP	SUPPLE-MENTS THAT HELP	HERBS THAT HELP	ALSO HELPS
Help your hair by incorporating in your diet a lot of vegetables and protein. Wheat germ (oil or flakes), Blackstrap, Molasses, Brewer's yeast, Seeds and nuts, Avocados. Food good for hair: all greens, carrots, green peppers, bananas, strawberries, apples, peas, onions, eggs, cucumbers, sprouts, unsaturated fat, especially olive oil. Avoid saturated fat and junk food.	EFA oils, B complex with B6, biotin and inositol, Vitamin C, Vitamin E, Zinc, CoQ10, Kelp, Copper, Silica, L-Cysteine, L-Methionine.	Sage tea rinse, Horsetail.	Brush hair upside down. Massage the scalp every day. Use alcohol-free products. Wash hair in warm, not hot water. Rinse in cool water. Rinse with cider vinegar or lemons. For added hair shine, try coconut oils, and to brighten hair color, use Chamomile. Avoid tabacco, alcohol, and caffeine. Occasionally use natural home products, like mayonnaise and olive oil to condition hair cuticles.

LEG AND MUSCLE CRAMPS

Muscle malfunctions are often the result of vitamin and mineral deficiencies. They are very often associated with loss of electrolyte minerals. Bountiful, healthy diets have been very successful in strengthening the body against nutrient shortages.

Symptoms: Spasms of the leg muscles, unexplained cramps.

Causes: Deficiency of calcium, potassium and other electrolytes; vitamin C deficiency causing poor collagen formation; food allergies and chronic exercise over-training.

FOODS THAT HELP	SUPPLEMENTS THAT HELP	HERBS THAT HELP	ALSO HELPS
Eat plenty of leafy greens, citrus fruit, brown rice, sprouts, broccoli, tomatoes, green peppers, bananas, beans and legumes, whole grains, dried fruit, sea vegetables, molasses, nuts, seafood. Drink green shakes. Avoid sugars and processed foods.	Kelp, Calcium, Magnesium, Vitamin E, Potassium, Silica, B complex plus extra B1 and niacin, Vitamin C, Vitamin D, CoQ10, Lecithin granules, Multivitamins and minerals, Zinc, Brewer's yeast.	Alfalfa, Dong quai, Elderberry extract, Gingko biloba, Horsetail grass, Valerian root.	Massage legs; elevate feet to stimulate circulation. Take a couple days of rest from exercise each week. Apply hot and cold alternating compresses to the area to ease pain and promote circulation. Get bi-monthly massages. Always warm-up, cool down and stretch thoroughly before and after exercise.

OBESITY (Being Overweight)

Being overweight is a condition of excess body fat that causes body weight to be over the ideal body weight for the person's height; obesity is classified as being 20 percent above that ideal. Weight management is a lifestyle, but many truly obese people do not eat any more food than their leaner counterparts.

Symptoms: Slow or dysfunctional metabolic rate, cravings for sugary foods, poor digestion and elimination, high blood pressure and cholesterol, depression, hunger.

Causes: There are many reasons, but underlying causes are not always well understood. Many obese people sustain sedentary lifestyles, follow yo-yo diets, have underactive thyroid, poor dietary habits, consume poor-quality foods and abide by irregular eating patterns (starve/binge).

FOODS THAT HELP	SUPPLEMENTS THAT HELP	HERBS THAT HELP	ALSO HELPS
Cut back on saturated fat but do not cut it out. Fat is not all bad; it's the chief source of energy for normal body function. Do not eat "empty calories," like processed and junk foods. Eat fruit and vegetables (raw). Do not go lower than 1000-1200 calories. Eat carbs, protein and fat at every meal. Choose foods rich in complex carbs (starch), also containing protein, such as beans and whole grains.	Multivitamins and minerals, Psyllium husks, Chromium picolinate, EFA oils, esp. flaxseed, primrose and salmon oil, Kelp, Lecithin granules, Spirulina, Vitamin C, Calcium, CoQ10, DHEA, L-Arginine, L-Ornithine, L-Lysine, L-Carnitine, L-Glutamine, L-Methionine, L-Phenylalanine, L-Tyrosine, Potassium, Vitamin B	Alfalfa, Corn-silk, Dandelion, Gravel root, Horsetail, Hydrangea, Hyssop, Juniper berries, Oat straw, Parsley, Thyme, Aloe vera juice, Butcher's broom, Cinnamon, Ginger, Green tea, Mustard seed, Cayenne.	Exercise most days of the week (a 3-mile walk can burn about 250 calories, depending on your weight). Lift weights to increase lean muscle mass and metabolism. (Muscle tissue uses up calories for energy. The greater the amount of muscle tissue you have, the more calories you can burn.) Try twelve-step programs, group therapy or individual therapy. Use meditation to reduce stress.

SMOKING AND RELATED PROBLEMS

Some studies say that each cigarette leeches eight minutes from your life; some say that a pack a day deletes one month from your life. Cigarettes have over 4,000 known poisons. Secondary or passive smoke and chewing tobacco are just as dangerous. Passive smoke reduces fertility, invites disease and ups your cancer risk—not to mention causing bad breath and smelly clothes. Smoking also disrupts insulin balance and metabolism.

Symptoms: Chronic bronchitis, constant hacking cough, difficulty breathing and shortness of breath, adrenal exhaustion, fatigue, poor circulation, high blood pressure, premature aging, dehydrated skin, stomach ulcers, low immunity, etc.

Causes: Stress, disease, nicotine poisoning and addiction, hypoglycemia, dietary deficiencies, peer pressure and a host of social behaviors.

FOODS THAT HELP	SUPPLEMENTS THAT HELP	HERBS THAT HELP	ALSO HELPS
Fast on fresh fruit and vegetable juices to neutralize and clear the blood from nicotine. Then eat leafy green salads, lots of citrus fruit to promote body alkalinity. Include lots of vegetable protein. Eat yellow and deep-orange vegetables like carrots, pumpkins, squash and yams. Eat smaller meals, more frequently, to maintain blood sugar levels. Avoid junk foods.	CoQ10, Vitamin C, Vitamin B complex plus B-12 and folic acid, Vitamin E, Vitamin A and beta carotene, Zinc.	Cayenne pepper, Catnip, Hops, Lobelia, Skullcap, Valerian root, Dandelion root, Milk thistle, Ginger, Slippery elm.	Practice yoga and deep-breathing exercises that deliver more oxygen to the body and its organs. Try patch treatments, support groups and therapy. To help curb cravings, chew licorice root sticks, calms root or cloves. You must exercise to help blood sugar levels (insulin excretion) and to build and regulate metabolism. Regular workouts also ease food cravings.

VARICOSE VEINS (and Spider Veins)

Varicose veins develop when a defect in the vein wall causes damage to the valves, and the ensuing pressure results in bulging veins. Varicose veins are often due to the loss of tissue tone, muscle mass and weakening of vein walls, especially with age. (Women are four times more prone than men).

Symptoms: Swollen, bulging leg veins; thin, red, spider veins; muscle cramps.

Causes: Sedentary lifestyle, low-fiber diet, meat and dairy diet with too much refined food; deficiency of essential fatty acids (EFAs), excess weight or pregnancy, poor posture and circulation, long periods of standing or heavy lifting.

FOODS THAT HELP	SUPPLEMENTS THAT HELP	HERBS THAT HELP	ALSO HELPS
Eat only fresh foods with plenty of green salads and juices. Then follow a predominantly vegetarian, high-fiber diet. Include seafood, beans, whole grains, brown rice, and lots of raw fruit. Take lecithin granules, brewer's yeast and wheat germ daily in nonfat yogurt. Reduce dairy products, fried food, prepared and red meat, saturated fat. Avoid salty, sugary and caffeinated foods.	CoQ10, EFA oils, Vitamin C, Vitamin E, Brewer's yeast, Lecithin granules, Multivitamin complex, Vitamin A and beta carotene, Vitamin B complex plus extra B6, Vitamin D plus calcium and magnesium.	Butcher broom, Gingko biloba, Gotu kola, Hawthorn berries, Horse chestnut, White oak bark tea (soak legs in it).	Bike, walk, run, stairclimb as much as possible to increase circulation and strengthen tissues. Elevate the legs during rest. Massage feet and legs regularly Go barefoot or wear flat sandals. Take mineral salts baths. Apply aloe vera gel. Do not use knee-high hosiery. In advanced or painful cases, surgery will help.

WATER RETENTION (Bloating and Edema)

Water retention is often caused by insufficient water consumption. Dieting, diet pills, diuretics, hormonal imbalances and over-exercising also cause this condition. If the body does not have sufficient water, it retains more water to compensate. Moreover, you lose vital electrolyte minerals (sodium, chloride, potassium, magnesium and calcium), which may cause fatigue or dizziness.

Symptoms: Swelling of hands, feet, ankles and stomach; PMS symptoms; headache, bloating and constipation.

Causes: Humid environment, chronic perspiration, excess protein, various infections, hypothyroidism, most premenstrual symptoms, protein and B-complex deficiency, hormonal changes, food allergies, air flight, obesity, lack of exercise.

FOODS THAT HELP	SUPPLEMENTS THAT HELP	HERBS THAT HELP	ALSO HELPS
Fasting flushes excess water. Reduce salt intake. Avoid junk foods. Drink at least 6 to 8 glasses of bottled water daily for free-flowing functions which help appetite suppression and elimination. Eat fresh raw foods to flush out excess water. Eat green salads every day, with cucumbers, parsley and celery.	Free-form amino acids, B-complex, Calcium, Magnesium, Silica, Bromelain, Garlic caps, Kelp, Potassium, Vitamin C, Vitamin E.	Alfalfa, Cornsilk, Butcher's broom, Dandelion root, Horsetail, Juniper berries, Parsley, Marsh mallow.	Drink at least 8-10 glasses of water each day, and more if you exercise regularly. Try steam baths or saunas but rehydrate immediately. Exercise regularly.

Scary diet story 11

Dating, for us, was like a calculus class. We had to manipulate, plan and time our dates in order to avoid the bitchy starvation phase of a diet, the active food orgy or the laxative relief phase. We would actually diet down for a date, with a specific day and time in mind.

Once, Shane was really anticipating an outing with a well-known personality. It was easy for her to "diet for him." But she had a minor food crisis: Should she eat before their dinner date and be able to pick at her meal in a ladylike way, or should she chance eating at the restaurant and risk a potential food frenzy? By then, dog food smelled good to us, so it was a difficult choice.

Of course, Shane lost the pounds and kept her stomach flat waiting for the "D day," the last diet day prior to her long-awaited date. But, unfortunately, she does not remember details about her date, their conversation, the atmosphere. Needless to say, though, Shane can vividly recall what she ordered (a whole lot) and just how everything tasted from that magical menu. The only thing Shane really remembers clearly about this great guy is what he told her after she polished off her third course. "I wish your eyes would light up for <u>me</u> the way they just did for your entrée," he said. There had been absolute adoration and love in her eyes. I don't think they dated again.

Scary diet story 12

"An apple a day keeps the doctor away," right? Well, we took poetic license with the phrase and transformed it into: "An apple a day keeps the FAT away." So we tried to follow that mutated promise and committed to eating an apple a day. That is, we ate exactly ONE apple a day—and nothing else! But then, we ate two on the second diet day, etc. Pretty soon, the number of apples correlated to the amount of days we followed this nifty meal plan. On the tenth day we ate ten apples. And on it went. It finally looked as though we were tiny lawnmowers, eating typewriter-style, in tidy rows—left to right. When we would get to the apple core, it would be like swallowing the worm in a tequila bottle. Down went the seeds, the stem and all. Surprisingly, we didn't have apple blossoms coming out of our ears.

Then came the twentieth day. Twenty apples. We could practically juice them with just our tongue and teeth. By this point, we could name the pesticides sprayed on the fruit, the soil they grew from, the compost used, even the cologne used by the apple handlers! By then, we were very frail, but talented, apple connoisseurs.

Chapter 7

The Barbis' get-gorgeous guide

Real beauty begins with inner health. Harmony and balance tend to show up first in your hair and skin since they are the two biggest telltale signs of real health. (Other signs manifest in the state of your teeth, bones and nails.). Since the body will not tolerate acids from a poor diet, or chemicals (it neutralizes them with alkali from those five places). Some people's genes will favor one or two but sacrifice the others. In pregnancy this occurs because the body will take from those five non-vital places to feed the baby. While it took us a long time to decipher this phenomenon, we have discovered that sickness, unhappiness, bad diets, smoking, doing drugs or eating lots of junk food all affect the inside of you, first. By the time you see traces of these poor habits show up on the outside, they have already done some internal damage.

On the other hand, once you adopt a nutritious food plan for life and begin exercising regularly, you are ready to tackle all of the other subtle nuances of beauty. Once you have mastered your health, then it's time to follow our guide to a truly gorgeous and healthy life, which always starts from the inside out.

Cosmic thoughts on cosmetics

We only wear makeup when we work. At home, we use homemade cleansers like apricot oatmeal scrubs or natural soaps that are pH balanced and perfume-free. We make honey face masks and use lemon as an astringent once a week, or so. (Sometimes a swim in the ocean does all of the above, and then the energy and feelings of wellness from the water exercise make your skin glow.)

We stick to natural makeup tricks for special dates and appearances in order to enhance our features—not change them. We believe that the three most important cosmetic categories affect:

- *the color of your skin,*
- *your eyes,*
- *your lips.*

Controversial to say the least, we do believe in maintaining a light, sun-kissed tan when possible. We heartily enjoy feeling 20 minutes of natural sunshine relax our body and mind. We think that Mother Nature is the best cosmetic.

To fake a natural tan, you can use a harmless sunless tanner (there are so many kinds available right now!), or try a light powder bronzer, which does not change the skin color, but adds highlights without clogging the pores. You can contour the face with a powder bronzer; a light brush above the cheekbones lengthens your face and jaw. Apply a light brush under the cheekbones to accentuate them; tracing under the jaw line provides a more pronounced jaw line.

Next are the eyes: The most important part of shaping your face is creating the slop of the eyebrows. We only pluck stray hairs from underneath the arch and start at the temples to pull the eyes outward. Most experts say that the eyebrow should stop at a 45-degree angle from the end of your eyes and should start straight up from the inside of your eye. If you do not naturally have dark eyebrows and want them darker, use a shade lighter than your mascara and brush eyebrows upward with a dry mascara brush. Then use a shade darker than your hair for mascara application; only brush the outer lashes and make sure there are no clumps. (We don't outline our eyes unless we're filming or shooting.) If you must further enhance your eyes, put a light brown shadow on the outer lids of both the top and bottom, close to the lashes, with a brown smudge.

Lips are an invitation to the rest of you. We do not recommend outlining lips since it seems to flatten them. On those rare makeup days, we use a coral or natural gloss, then dab a shimmery light or white powder on the upper cupids and the very middle of the lower lip only. This gives the illusion of fuller lips. If you already sport a sexy pout, add Vaseline on top of the earth-tone lipstick in order to brighten your lips. (While we haven't asked men for their opinion on the subject, we happen to think red lips are an eyesore.)

Always do your makeup in good light. Lighting from above (even sunlight) or from underneath will distort your view. Even a good makeup job can be mistaken for a 'Frankenstein Face' due to horrible lighting. Plus, makeup should be removed as soon as possible. Makeup removers usually have chemicals or perfumes that are just as irritating as the makeup itself. We use natural removers like a mixture of apricot oil, coconut oil and avocado. We use a Q-tip around the lash area, then blot our eyes lightly with a warm washcloth. Use a natural astringent, like witch hazel, without alcohol, to remove makeup residue after you wash your face. We also wait a few minutes before applying night cream or moisturizer: we want our skin to breathe.

We firmly believe in the following statement: hair can make or break your style. Certainly, you may have a preference for something different than you already have, but always get close to what looks natural. For example, if you have curly dark hair, leave the curls, but, maybe, loosen them. Apply natural henna to the hair to bring out highlights. We think that the best blondes are summer blondes with highlights. The most natural way we lighten our hair is with lemon, vinegar and chamomile tea. If you have straight hair, like ours, make it fuller by blow-drying the head upside down and brushing the hair forward towards the forehead. (Sparkling water and other carbonated beverages will also boost lift when added to the hair.)

Put natural gel, just on the roots, when blow-drying to make your hair fuller. We prefer natural shampoos, like the ones we use on our horses. This natural horse shampoo makes hair mane-like, healthy and thick. We condition our hair after a lot of ocean or pool swimming, with natural avocado or mayonnaise; too much conditioning makes our hair limp. We always put a very thin layer of olive oil on our hair before swims, saunas or any sun exposure, as a preventive measure and to ensure tangle-free tresses.

Haircuts are absolutely vital. We cut our hair, at least half an inch every six weeks; our hair grows like weeds, which means it's healthy; but long hair is hard to style, and it often looks flat. However, a great cut makes the hair heavier at the ends, prevents split ends, aids growth and makes you feel like a million bucks! We never blow-dry or lighten our ends. If you must use a hair dryer, set it on cool.

If you want to achieve hair length with more body, layering might be the way to go. Research for a good hairdresser like you would for a doctor, and check out his work in person. If you want an inch cut off, make sure it is not one inch three times over! And do not offer to be a model for a hairdresser debut unless you are exceptionally brave and daring. Unless you're shopping in Paris, it'll look too "avant garde" to be seen with the "Star Trek Special" at your neighborhood grocery store.

It is natural to lose about 25 hairs a day. The more you curl, blow-dry, dye or bleach your hair, though, the more you damage it. We think that natural bristle hairbrushes are the best because rubber and steel brushes cause breakage. For straight long hair—like ours—finger brushing is best. (Remember: long hair is old hair, which needs special care.)   Also, use large-pronged combs and start combing from the bottom up. Never rip tangles out; "wiggle" them out in pieces instead, starting from the ends. Vinegar is a good detangler (in small amounts). We do not wash our hair more often than every other day; wet hair is vulnerable and breaks easily.

We think that in small, protected increments, the sun complements your skin. On the other hand, the sun damages hair by draining oil and destroying pigmentation. The best sun block for your hair is a hat. We have mentioned that chamomile tea is a hair lightener, but chamomile oil is much stronger. Brunettes can use coffee rinses, and redheads can use red zinger tea to highlight their heads.

If you want a natural-looking perm, try this trick at the beach or by the pool when the hair is damp. Twist small sections of your hair in spongy rollers (the smaller the curler—the tighter the look) and "bake" it naturally in the sun. This will give you a lasting perm without the damage of a chemical perm. And for the dreaded "green aftermath" from chlorine pools, crush six aspirins into warm water, comb through, then rinse. One of our top tricks when the hair is oily, and you don't have time to wash it? Add baby powder and finger-brush.

What is right for you?

Saunas are good for hair, skin and overall relaxation. Akin to a facial, dry heat opens pores, clears the skin of impurities and prevents blemish build-up. Especially if you are prone to dryness, put a light sunflower or carrot oil on your face or hair to act like a hot oil treatment. Be careful of too much oil, of course. It's heavy and takes many washes to eradicate completely (try dampening the ends with a light coat instead).

Aromas, or natural perfumes, always set the mood. Whether you want to feel sexy and energized, romantic or mysterious—you can say it all with scent. Natural aromas we love, are: rose oil, sandalwood oil, lavender extract, almond oil, citrus oils, honeysuckle, and apple blossom extract and jasmine oil. Baking soda is also an effective natural deodorant. (Remember not to put perfume on before sunbathing—it's a skin irritant.)

The condition of your nails—on your hands or feet—provides a major clue to the condition of your body. Healthy nails are strong and smooth and should always be simply and naturally adorned. Ridged or grooved nails may indicate liver imbalances or calcium depletion. Pale or discolored nails indicate poor blood flow, possible anemia or a metabolic dysfunction. Healthy nails are not brittle, flaky or easily broken.

We use lemon to lighten and polish our nails. We cringe at some of the expensive "claws" women invest in today. Polish should be removed every few weeks, so your nails can breathe, or they turn brittle or yellow and sometimes become infected. Stick with clear, peach or skin tones, and forget the fancy nail extensions. Instead, put that money toward a pair of good running shoes. You'll get much better returns on your beauty investment!

Dressing to look sleek, chic and LEAN is an expert area for the Barbi Twins... How many times, after a binge, were we told about an interview the following morning! David Copperfield, move over! Naturally, dark colors are more slimming, and black hose, if appropriate, can be the most stylish camouflage. But in the summertime, we often stray toward navy blue or tonal earth hues.

Plain, monochromatic colors tend to create one long, unbroken style line from head to toe; minimize prints except for thin vertical stripes that train the eye to go up and down (think pin stripes). We think dark dresses hide "extras" better than skirts, whereas sweaters and bulky shirts make you look like you're hiding imperfections. Wear only one bright color to break up your "dark veils:" either shoes, a blouse under a blazer, or a scarf around your neck or shoulders. Although styles for the last two seasons have leaned toward very long skirts and dresses, a little black dress never goes out of style—especially if you have great legs.

Awesome accessories, to us, are a watch and a backpack, to complement our jeans and boots. When we do dress up, however, we minimize all of the little extras (on twins, especially, too much of anything looks tacky). We wear simple belts with jeans, and we prefer small hoop earrings. Our necklaces are simple gold or silver chains with, maybe, a cross. We only wear thin rings that were given to us by close friends or family, and only on special occasions. We love wearing our hair up in a twist with simple barrettes.

One question that we are continually asked is how we would dress up for a dream date. It is simply ... simple! Light makeup (with a slight tan), hair up in a twist, a classic black dress, black pumps (or plain dinner shoes), a small black purse, no accessories and plain stockings. Whether it is makeup, nails, hair, dress or accessories, less is more (no pun intended). More appealing!

We want to make a special note here, at the end of our beauty guide. Simply put, you can always enhance your physical appearance, even if you're not at your goal weight. You cannot buy health, however; you must earn it. Mother Nature does not make unattractive people, only bad habits do! We guarantee this: take any person and help her become her fittest, happiest and best, and she will be beautiful. Just look at someone who is in love. They glow with inner spirit and energy. Beauty is a by-product of your discipline and hard-earned health. This never fails; it is a lifelong warranty, gifted by God.

Scary diet story 13

A trip to the dentist is something that normal people dread. Not us. Visiting our dentist signifies an enforced diet—a real pain in the mouth—and tells us that our teeth, luckily, did not bear the brunt of our eating disorders. (Considering the amount of junk food, sugars and vomiting we did for years, we could have massacred our mouths. Lucky for us, we still have strong, healthy teeth and gums. Go figure.) Another reason we love the dentist is that we have looked into wiring our jaws closed to enforce a fast. Again—lucky for us—doctors thought we were too thin for such radical procedures.

One of my fondest dental memories (I have a few!) was when I had my wisdom teeth pulled. Every single person I knew lost weight because it hurt to eat. Yahoo! For once, it was even safe to leave leftovers in the refrigerator because I knew that I'd be in no shape to scarf them up with stitches in my mouth.

Right after surgery, I was driven home with my throbbing mouth packed with gauze. (Remember the overstuffed, groggy chipmunk look?) But as soon as I hit the kitchen, the leftover cookies filling the room greeted me like a cheap potpourri. At first, the sight made me ill. Then, slowly, the smell made me feel better. I imagined the cookies gently massaging my mouth. I didn't remember any rough edges. And then I remembered the dentist ordering soft foods and juices only. Soft foods, huh? In seconds, I was smashing the cookies, mixing them with milk and water and creating a sweet, puree paste on the kitchen table. Like a cocaine addict, I smeared the mixture into my aching mouth. Every last crumb.

I think I could have been in the Guinness Book of World Records as the only person who <u>gained</u> weight after a wisdom tooth extraction. Well, make that two. Shane loved my invention, too.

Scary diet story 14

Through the years, we devised ways to stop our feeding frenzies, which could have continued all night long. Even as prepubescents, we concocted ways to conquer forbidden foods; locked doors had hinges and notes posted on the refrigerator ("Do Not Be A Pig," for instance) made us squeal with laughter.

Then we came upon the secret to our senses: make the food inedible—make it taste awful. We learned this at a restaurant when a waitress wore too much cheap perfume, and it almost ruined our appetite. Hmmm. We would get set to binge with our aroma pick-of-the-week beside us. At about the time we decided we should feel full, we'd pour the pretty little scent on the remaining food. (Later, we learned to use dish soap because our dishes started smelling like a whorehouse.)

The tricks stopped working—alas, they always do. One night, a few months later, we did the dishes after dinner and threw away the extra food with dish soap squirted on top, as usual. Two hours later, our stomachs grumbled for a midnight snack, but no stores were open and we'd already eaten everything in the pantry and freezer. Without hesitation, we went through the trash like narc dogs on a mission. All the food was still intact; there was just a little "soap glaze" that didn't seem to permeate the twilight treat… no big deal. A little splash; a little sprinkle, and it was back to its original state. Sick… but delicious!

Chapter 8

The Barbis' exercise guide

We discovered, at a very early age, that almost any type of exercise offers multiple rewards. Born prematurely—we weighed only three pounds each at birth—we were plagued with various illnesses as children. Shane especially suffered because she was born with asthma, and had terrible attacks during her early years. Through a love of horses and sports, we were able to overcome our physical weaknesses. In fact, Shane gave up her asthma medications in high school and joined the track team. She eventually broke a six-minute mile—a school record—without a single wheeze!

Our father taught skiing, and we were always encouraged to go outside and play. In addition to skiing frequently and being on the school swim team, we regularly played basketball and softball, ice skated, roller skated and took ballet and tap dance classes. Exercise, we have learned, helps get kids off the couch and helps them experience a sense of competition and fair play. Sports are a great social source for children.

In addition to the purely physical and social effects of exercise, research shows that regular exercise strengthens the heart, lungs and other organs, helps water retention, fatigue and anxiety, lowers depression and eases stress, improves posture and body image and helps prevent a host of illnesses, including diabetes, asthma and high blood pressure.

The Surgeon General's Report says that the minimal exercise requirement to maintain general health is 20-30 minutes of exercise, three days per week. (Of course, we say that's sufficient only if you're climbing out of a hospital bed!) Beyond these minimal health guidelines, most experts recommend more weekly activity. For weight loss (or maintenance) and optimal fitness benefits, we suggest 45-60 minutes of aerobic exercise most days of the week, in addition to weight lifting (body sculpting—whatever you want to call it) three or four times a week. Always warm-up, cool down and stretch after every workout to prevent injuries and increase performance. As with anything else, variety is the key to success and adherence.

To exercise aerobically means to work out "with oxygen," indicating any sustained, moderate activity that keeps heart rate raised and steady over an extended period of time. Examples of aerobic activities include walking, hiking and swimming. Aerobic (or "cardio") exercises can last anywhere from 10 minutes to several hours, depending on your fitness level. They create a demand on the heart and lungs to deliver oxygen to the bloodstream, where food is metabolized as energy (fuel).

An anaerobic workout (without oxygen) typically refers to stop-and-start activities that require quick bursts of energy followed by a lull—weight lifting, tennis and wind sprints, for instance. As in aerobic exercise, the fuel that makes an anaerobic activity possible comes from glycogen (calories stored as by-products of the food we eat), which is provided mainly by carbohydrates and fat. (Proteins are used very sparingly as available energy—they are too busy repairing and building muscle cells.) The fuel for high-intensity anaerobic activity typically runs out after a few seconds or minutes, whereas aerobic fuel can last much longer.

Most dieters believe that they only need aerobic exercise to lose weight. This is not exactly true. You need both kinds: aerobic for heart, lungs and fat burning; and anaerobic for stronger muscles and bones, and for speeding up your metabolism. There are also conflicting opinions about the most effective exercise mode and workout intensity. Most experts claim that extended periods of continuous (but not bone-breaking) and moderate cardio exercise burn more fat. In fact, training at very high aerobic intensities adds the anaerobic element (so you may not burn as much fat per session), but you still burn lots of calories and rev up your metabolism simultaneously.

Our favorite fat-fighting exercises

This list of aerobic activities is culled from our many tried-and-true routines. We have old stand-byes and new favorites, but here we rate each activity based on how effective we think it is; in addition to how efficient it has proved to be for blasting calories. No matter what exercise routine you choose, be careful not to over-exercise and not to cause injury to your ligaments. Use protective gear. For almost any exercise involving legs, we recommend using knee wraps so that not to favor certain muscles while exploiting the others; moreover, they will support you knees, and will protect them from injury. As far as the type of exercise goes, your own individual preferences and athletic skills will determine which mode works best for you. As you will see on the following pages, your own personal body type also may play a role in what activity helps you achieve the quickest (and most permanent) results:

1. *Running (the most intense form is jogging on uneven terrain or soft sand);*
2. *Kickboxing, Tae Bo, boxing;*
3. *Cross-country skiing (lower and upper body workout);*
4. *Stair-climbing or stepping and elliptical training;*
5. *Biking (high-intensity mountain biking or Spinning classes);*
6. *In-line skating (rollerblading);*
7. *Aerobic dance (high intensity);*
8. *Power walking (hike up hills with a weighted backpack);*
9. *Swimming (use harder strokes—back stroke, butterfly);*
10. *Racquetball (play singles court sports, and keep moving).*

Weight lifting for total health

Strength training is for people who want to build muscle, sculpt their body, improve appearance and posture, kick-start their metabolism, help prevent injuries, improve body composition (read—"less fat") and help build stronger bone connections. In fact, one of the most important reasons to lift weights regularly—and it's never too late to start—is to build denser bones in order to help prevent osteoporosis.

As muscles get stronger, so do bones. Here are some osteoporosis facts that may motivate you to lift your first set of free weights:

- *80 percent of all osteoporosis sufferers are women;*
- *Half of all women will get the disease at some point in their lives;*
- *You achieve peak bone mass by the age of 30, and it dwindles from there;*
- *Strict dieters and people with eating disorders are at much higher risk;*
- *Caucasians, smokers and very small-boned people are at higher risk.*

What's the best strategy?

Now that you know you should strength-train regularly, how do you start? To sculpt muscle definition and improve functional strength, the American College of Sports Medicine recommends lifting three sets of 8-15 repetitions per exercise. And most experts suggest choosing three different exercises per body part to get optimal results, as well as lifting weights for different parts of the body at least three days per week. Al-

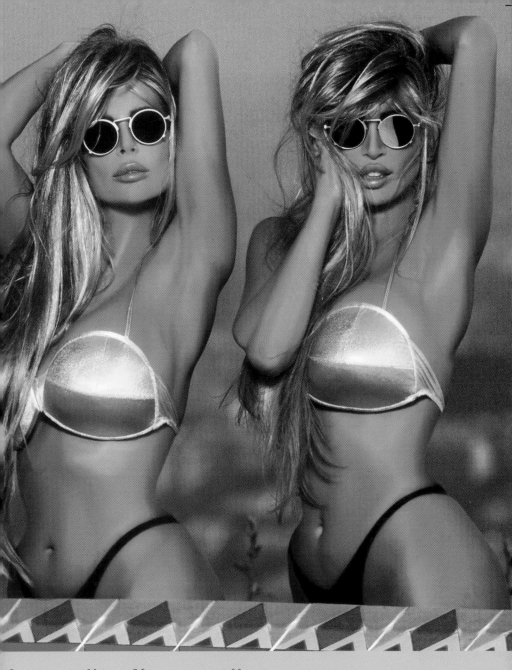

Sia at 145 lbs., Shane at 148 lbs.

At this time we were following the protein diet and exercising eight hours daily. The diet was ~iling because we had done it too many times before. Instead of dehydrating us, as the pro~ ~n diet usually does, it made us bloat. We binged because we were upset about the failing ~et. We also started taking laxatives in huge amounts and throwing up our meals. Greg ~orman, a true master of photographic art, had us raise our arms to create an illusion of thin ~aists and get rid of the fat rolls, and hid our big hips and legs behind the pool.

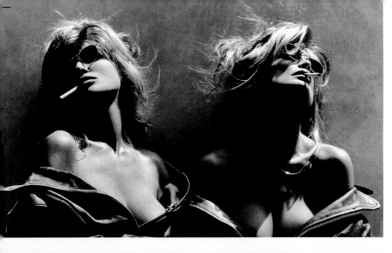

Though I was alwa
health conscious, I
tried smoking to lose
weight. Shane alway
said she'd rather be fa
and healthy than be a
smoker. I lost weight
but I too wanted to
healthy, so I quit.

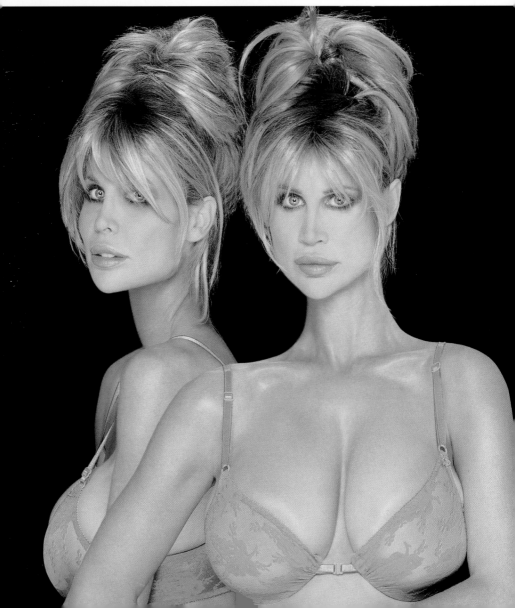

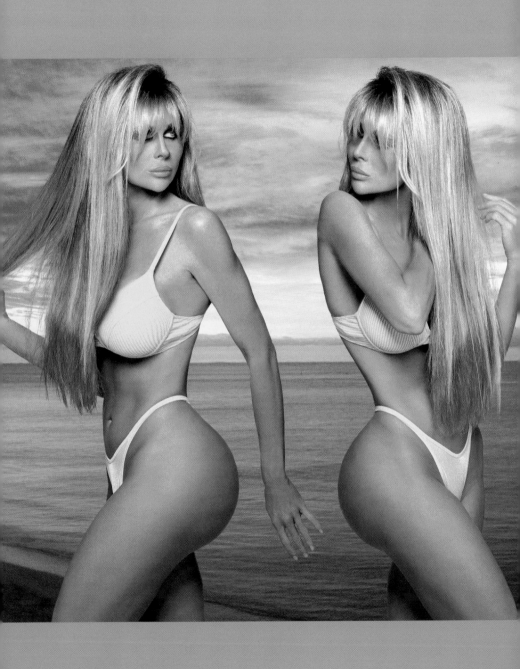

"The Cowgirl."
This is how
I like to dress.

~Sia

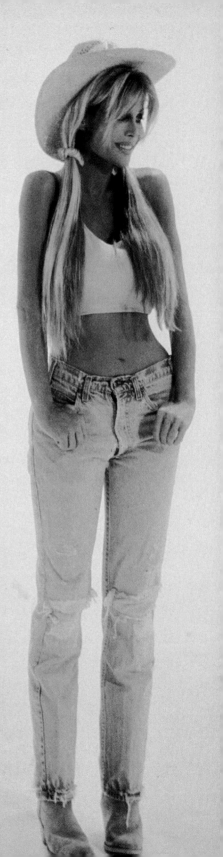

(Shane) Barbi marries Ken (Ken Wahl, award~winning actor from the hit TV series Wise Guy).

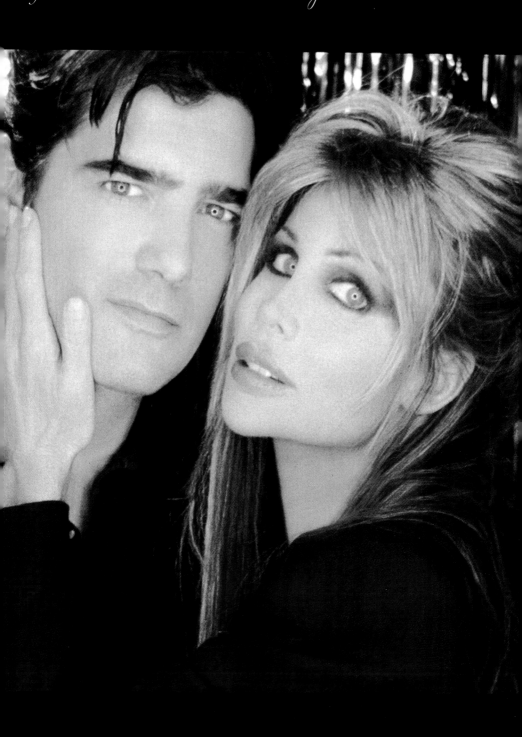

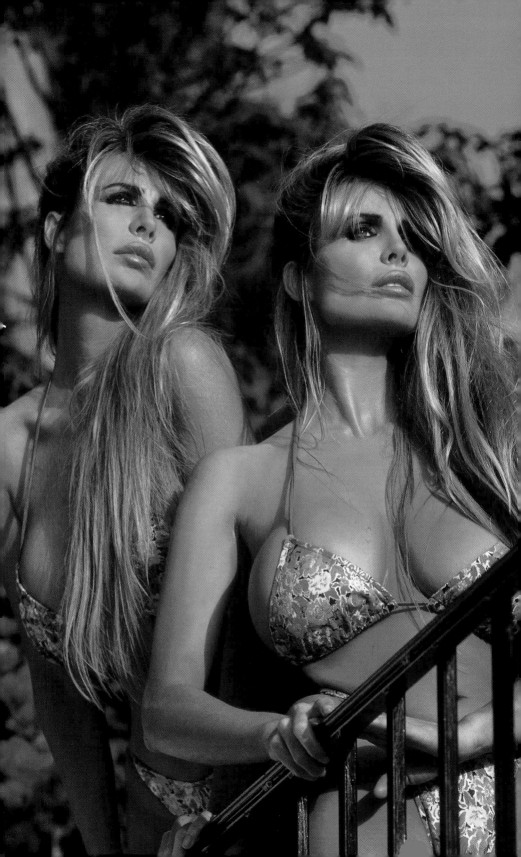

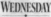
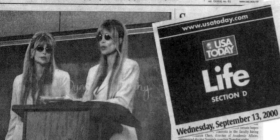
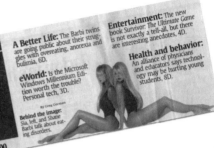
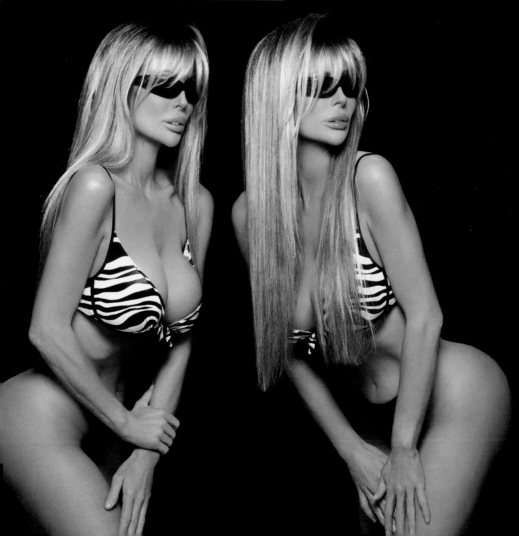

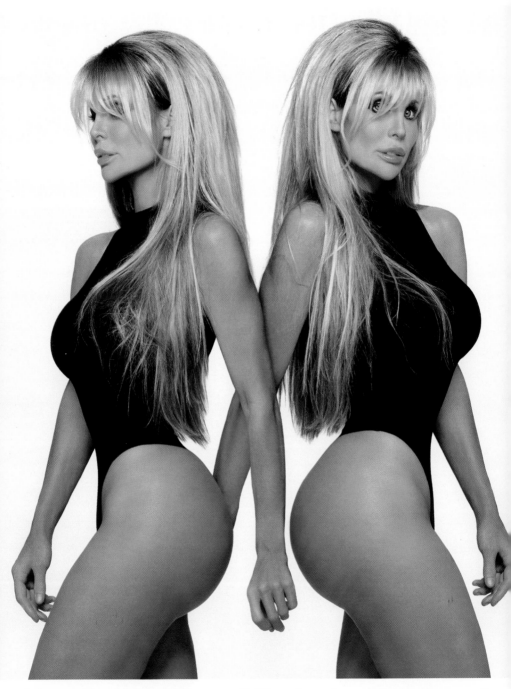

There is nothing wrong with beauty itself. But when it becomes the main focus, an obsessi it becomes an addiction. Therefore, beauty should not be a goal, but rather a by~produc daily efforts to achieve the state of radiant health. Weight, too, should not be a goal, but rat a by~product of right living.

~She

ways skip a day of lifting in between sessions to rest and repair your active muscles.

It is best to ask a trainer about your intensity level and weight amount if you're just starting out. We've worked up to lifting fairly heavy weights three to four times a week.

Do not overdo; when you're ready to increase the weight or try a new exercise, go slowly and up your weight in light increments to avoid injury. Intense muscle soreness is a warning that you may have pushed too hard the day before. Stretching after each lifting session will help relieve soreness; massage and a warm bath with salts will also relieve symptoms of delayed onset of muscle soreness.

Most avid body builders prefer resistance training with free weights (dumbbells) instead of the resistance machines found in health clubs nationwide. For women who just want to "tone up," any form of weights (tubing, body bars or exercise bands) will suffice, as long as you're lifting right. (There are excellent how-to videos on the market today.)

A term we've become fond of is "peaking." It means going beyond your normal intensity range in either aerobics or weight training sessions. We usually know we're "peaking" if we start sweating profusely or can't catch our breath. We've experimented so much and know our bodies so well, that we know when we're peaking. But many exercisers do not.

Many active people depend on measuring their performance by taking their heart rate before and after exercise—especially during cardio activity. A heart rate monitor is extremely accurate, but it's expensive, and does not allow you to become accustomed to your own body fluctuations. (It's like a therapist telling me WHY I over-ate.) It's best to spend our time focusing on solutions. Below, we've listed three easy methods to measure your workout intensity. The third method is the most accurate and complete, also allowing you to measure your own recovery rate after the workout. Your recovery heart rate is a significant indicator of your cardiovascular fitness:

Method 1—talk test
If you can hold a breathy conversation while exercising, you are working at an efficient level. If you cannot hold a conversation, you should lessen the intensity. If, on the other hand, you can converse easily during a workout, then increase intensity to see better results. (It should never be really easy to chat with your treadmill neighbor!)

Method 2—perceived exertion test
This scale demands that you rate your own exercise intensity depending on how difficult it feels to you intrinsically. (This is a great way to get

to know your own body, so practice consistently.) Consider "O" as no workload and "10" is working so hard you cannot continue for more than a few seconds. Keep self-checking your intensity during each session: experts say the most effective calorie-burning ranges fall between 6, 7 and 8. But you should fluctuate throughout each session.

Method 3—heart rate test

If you have a heart rate monitor, the gadget does these calculations for you. If not, become adept at taking your own neck or wrist pulse:

a) First thing in the morning, take your MORNING PULSE for one minute and remember the number. (The lower the number—in the 50s, 60s or 70s—the fitter you are.) Then, subtract your age from the number 220. (If you're 20 years old, subtracting 20 from 220 = 200.)

b) If you know your most effective training heart rate zone, you can boost cardiovascular health and blast body fat. To determine intensity via heart rate during a cardio workout, take that 200 number (above) and multiply it by .70 and .85. Now try to keep your workout pulse in those fat-burning zones for most of your exercise sessions. (For example, when that 20-year-old takes a neck or wrist pulse during exercise, she should effectively try to stay between 140 and 170 beats-per-minute for best body results.)

c) Recovery heart rate. This is how long it takes for your heartbeat to return to normal. After your workout, keep walking slowly and take a one-minute pulse. Register that recovery number, and see how close it comes to the MORNING PULSE you took above (see (a) above). The fitter you are, the quicker you will recover. (Be sure to take your pulse immediately after each workout to get an accurate baseline.)

Exercise is as important as a balanced, moderate diet. They work synergistically to achieve optimal physical and mental health.

Best moves for your body type

There are basically three types of bodies and many crossover combinations of these predominant types: the endomorph, ectomorph and mesomorph. Most people tend to be mostly one type with some attributes of one other. See if you can identify your shape here:

An endomorph is usually shorter, strong and curvy and tends to gain weight easily, especially around her hips and butt. Her exercise priority is to burn lots of cardio calories to control body fat, and to strength-train regularly, in order to maximize lean muscle tissue. Good exercises for endomorphs are power walking, cross-country skiing and body sculpting classes.

An ectomorph is usually taller and thin, and has a hard time gaining curves or muscle mass. She probably has an efficient metabolism, but needs to stretch regularly and work on building muscle through sports and leisure activities. Good exercises for endomorphs are lifting with heavier weights, yoga and all sorts of court sports.

A mesomorph lies somewhere between the endomorph and the ectomorph, but has a more athletic physique. Mesomorphs are of medium build, and of average weight. Good exercises for this body type include balance training, martial arts, stair-climbing and resistance training.

Your body structure can be a combination of any of the three types; therefore, determining your exercise routine according to your body type is not an exact science. Don't avoid doing your favorite activity just because we have not listed it here—you are the best judge of what works and what does not.

Yoga and stretching

Unfortunately, we were the kind of exercisers who could not be bothered with stretching, bowling, golf, or anything that that did not make us sweat profusely. (No sweat? Forget it!) But then after a long day of horseback riding, we registered this epiphany: when you jump a horse, that jump is only a part of the course. There's the striding, the take-off, the jump itself, then the follow-through. It's like a chain or an assembly line. And the better your preparation, the better the jump will be. This variety prevents the horse from going sour or getting bored. The horse uses different muscles for different jumps—which prevents overuse injuries—and all jumps will benefit if he doesn't do the same old thing each time.

And so, the same thing goes for us. Performing yoga, stretching, balance training, T'ai Chi and extra-curricular exercises will tone you and prepare you for a better, safer and more enduring core workout. Stretching (and yoga) also help develop muscles and protect them from injury. Every muscle contracting during an exercise should be stretched afterwards to create a balanced workout.

Yoga and other eastern philosophies stress the importance of proper breathing, and many fitness experts claim that breathing itself is an exercise. Proper breath-work helps bring more oxygen through the bloodstream and delivers it to your active muscles. The best advice we can give is do not hold your breath during any exercise. Breathe evenly, deeply and consistently. Deep breathing can actually be a form of meditation, good for long, drawn-out endurance events. Breath-work during yoga helps balance the body mentally, physically and, for some, spiritually. Yoga can create a more fulfilling workout, allowing you to relax from stress and better prioritize your life. Yoga can be extremely strenuous, too, depending on the instructor. It is as easy as you make it. It is as tough as you push it.

Your "no-time" exercise plan

Okay, here are some good excuses: I cannot afford a gym. I'm too busy. It's just too inconvenient. Gyms are dirty, too crowded, they are meat markets. Health clubs and YMCAs are not places for fat people; besides, they're not exciting enough. Running is bad for the knees and/or for a woman's reproductive system. Bikes are uncomfortable or dangerous, especially at night or in traffic. Swimming is nice if it is 85 balmy degrees outside, but there are creepy crawlers in the water! I do not want to sweat, ruin my make-up, or muss my hair. My legs hurt! Fitness trainers make me cry—they intimidate me—and working out is simply too depressing. Enough?

Yes, we've heard them all, and then some. You either want it or you don't. Please just start sweating, and we can intellectualize after your workout. When we ran marathons, we used every excuse in the world to stop, but found we were committed to the challenge. Overcoming the chattering negative voices in your head will allow you to fight FOR your body—and truly excel.

Make exercise a routine that you can stick with; home exercise is the most painless, time-efficient, convenient way to start a program. A jump rope is so simple, and yet so effective. (A 130-pound woman can burn 100 calories in 10 quickie minutes!) If you have a long set of steps in or near your home, hike them for 15 minutes while listening to your Walkman.

There were too many times, during on-location photo shoots, when we were forced to jump around in our tiny hotel bathroom. But we did it! Or we performed calisthenics in our hotel room. Push-ups, sit-ups and leg raises can be done just using the floor, the wall or any old chair. (We also love the "phone book trick." It's great for horseback riding: Bend knees slightly in a semi-squat and hold a phone book for as long as you can between your thighs.) Large plastic water bottles filled with water or sand make excellent free weights. Some people carry those weightless exercise bands to body-sculpt when they're on the road. Great! Anything can work if you focus on your muscles and stop making excuses. And you can stretch absolutely anywhere...

In-home exercise equipment—a treadmill, bike, and those fancy new elliptical trainers that go backwards—allow you to kill two birds with one dumbbell. Plus, you can exercise your body and your mouth (on the phone) in one shot. We have personally found that outdoor workouts are more motivating and feel more beneficial—especially for breathing and relaxation—but we frequently supplement these sessions with in-home workouts.

Other home-based moves

Use your bed
Lie facedown; hang off the side with torso toward the floor. Keep feet flat up against a wall, and slowly move the upper body up and down to strengthen your lower and middle back. Then, from the same position (bring torso up onto the bed tummy-down), alternate rear leg lifts to boost your butt. Then lie face-up on the bed flat with feet together and tummy tight. Thrust only your hips up as you squeeze your buttocks together (master the pelvic tilt). Do tummy crunches in bed for pure decadence.

The kitchen sink
Stand in front of the sink with feet at least two feet away from the base of the counter. With hands clutching the sink, perform counter push-ups with hands shoulder-distance apart. As you wash those dirty dishes, why not strap on a pair of 2-pound ankle weights and perform inner and outer thigh kicks?

Use books as weights
Stand up straight with feet about shoulder-width apart. Take a book in each hand and curl up to shoulders for biceps, then lift books straight out to the sides for shoulder raises. Then, extend both books overhead, bending your arms at the elbows, and lift and slowly lower the books to strengthen your triceps, that frustrating jiggly area in the back of your arm.

Use pets or kids ... gently
Play a version of tug of war, tag, fetch or hide-and-seek every single day. Maintain a semi-squat position to contract leg muscles and keep abs tight at all times. Bottom line is, there's always some activity that you can do which will keep your metabolism stoked, and your body - toned. You do not have to spend money on a gym membership or lose too much time commuting.

We get really angry with people who say derogatory things like: "Sure, Oprah can lose weight. She can afford her own gym, chef and personal trainer around the clock; I could lose it if I were that rich." Shame on them for saying that! Not only is Oprah a self-made success story, but she finds the time in her very hectic schedule for the most strenuous exercise routine. Focused winners like Oprah certainly did not BUY drive, discipline or desire; they cultivate those principles on their own. They work hard, wealthy or not. And so can you!

Best time to exercise

This is a big controversy, and there's no easy answer to the question. Some say mornings, some say midday or even after dinner. It depends on your personal preference and on what you want to accomplish, really. We like to do aerobics first thing in the morning when we have a clear head, when the day's pressures have not yet descended. We also like to lift weights or do aerobics classes before our biggest meal of the day, which is, often, lunch.

Sometimes long cardio hits at night are fun and we can really relax and train as long as we want. (Our best mega-workouts are usually done at night.). However, some nighttime exercisers are too revved up, for us to sleep after an evening session. And, then again, sometimes we dread midday workouts because we have to wait half the day to get it done.

A few exercise guidelines to live by, whatever time of day or night serves you best:

DON'T exercise on a totally full or empty stomach. You'll feel crampy and gassy if you've eaten a meal within 90 minutes of a tough workout. On the other hand, an empty stomach cannot fuel you properly for a long routine, either. (You'll go harder and longer with something light and nutritious in your system.) If you're hungry leading up to your workout, ingest some light calories at least one hour before your workout—a big glass of juice or a fruit salad might suffice—to keep your blood sugar steady and your workout energized.

Some people like to split up their routines and wake up to a long cardio workout. To give metabolism a double whammy, these people like to lift weights later on in the day. Just be sure to get at least 20 minutes of continuous exercise each time—whether it's straight aerobics, weights, or a combination of both. And always drink plenty of water before, during and after your routine.

There is a theory that dawn and dusk are the best times to exercise. Although it's a simplistic principle, we tend to agree. Whether it is the extra negative ions in the air at sunrise or the ambient backdrop of a setting sun, we have better workouts at these times. Morning workouts tend to flush the skin, heighten circulation, focus concentration and reduce bloat. Evening workouts often help us ease the stress of the day, help us wind down and give us the time to exercise longer and harder. There are fewer appointments to keep at the end of the day. Your body is also more flexible at night, so yoga and stretching classes are optimal in the PM. Then again, when we need to pour over contracts, memorize lines or use our mental muscle, a midday workout breaks up the stress and strain.

So, it really depends on your individual schedule, preferences and desires. But a recurring routine is important. After six months or so, it will become a habit. And then you are on your way to lifelong fitness.

Scary diet story 15

Dining out can be tricky when practicing the art of laxative abuse. If you don't time it perfectly, and orchestrate the evening's itinerary to the exact minute, things could get messy. One time, we received an invitation from a well-known celeb to dine at a fabulous health food restaurant. We thought that we could order anything because we had choreographed our laxative routine to discard any unwanted food. It was like winning a lottery—free calories. The evening was proceeding rather well, and we were actually having fun. That is, until Shane had a premature evacuation <u>urge</u>. (Urge is putting it very, very mildly.) She begged me to stand at the bathroom door to guarantee her privacy while she practiced her Lamaze-like technique on the bathroom floor. Time went by; her moaning began to worry me. The ungodly sounds continued for way too long; people approached the bathroom and quickly turned around. Tick, tick, tick. Twenty minutes later, she finally emerged. There was an alarming silence for a long moment. Then Shane cheerfully announced, "I'm hungry!" And the cycle began again…

Scary diet story 16

We are very clean and organized, which is part of our disease. We are so co-dependent that we like controlling other people's lives, relationships, cars, homes; you name it. After one tough photo shoot, we planned a big binge as a reward. To escape the Hollywood hoopla, we decided to visit a good friend in a remote area out of state. (I still remember that she had gift-wrapped a box of candy for us as a welcoming gift.)

After our friend went to sleep, Shane and I were still jumpy—and not from the difficult magazine shoot—but because we had that addictive pre-binge excitement. (There's nothing like it in the world.) We decided to clean our friend's kitchen cabinets — how could she possibly live in a house with so much untouched, forbidden food? It took about half the night to finish our chore.

If our friend had gotten up in the middle of the night to see what all the crinkling, crackling and giggling was about, she would have caught us, rancid food dribbling from our mouths, like a couple of stunned grazing deer, caught in the headlights of a car.

BUT: Our lovely friend woke up the next morning to the cleanest kitchen she had ever seen … and the emptiest! There were only a few boring cans of vegetables or soup left in the cupboards. But the surprise was on us: we were stunned when she said that some of those packaged cookies and crackers had been in her pantry for over five years! Our stomachs started to grumble.

Two months later, we received a gift in the mail from our out-of-state friend. It was a package of "dog chewies." She wrote a cute note saying, "How could you have missed these? They're delicious!" She obviously meant it as a joke, but we loved those beef-jerky things, quite a calorie-free treat for the adventurous Barbi Twins.

Chapter 9

Good and bad role models, support groups

We come from an athletic family who practiced consistent, conscientious eating habits. Through the years, we have frequently thought about our eating disorders, "Why us?" We believe now that our food obsessions and unhealthy body image were the manifestations of other dysfunctional patterns in our early lives. In our family, as in many others, alcohol and other abnormal reactions were used to "medicate" any turbulent situations instead of dealing with problems head-on. And so, we learned this behavior and turned to food as the means of escape.

It may seem cute and innocent to eat like a horse when you're young and spindly. Around puberty, however, when hormones kick in, and peer pressure raises its ugly head, that type of deportment is no longer adorable. There is so much pressure to be pretty, popular and thin for a young teen today.

With a nod toward the trends of the day and towards what's important to youth 2000, we think that it's sad that generation X-ers (and even younger kids) can identify and name international supermodels, but are stumped when naming foreign presidents or Prime ministers.

Probably better than most, however, we understand societal discrepancies. Let's ponder these disturbing questions: Who promotes models to sign multi-million dollar deals based on their physical beauty? And who purchases women's magazines, buys expensive cosmetics, and sets the overall trends that flaunt physical perfection? It's all about supply and demand. And it's all about women's market. If advertisers hawk their wares, and women buy their products by the dozens, why condemn a young, skinny model for promoting anorexia? The advertisers put her on that page (or screen) because they are paid to give women what they really want.

Then what happens? Instead of supporting each other—and coming to terms with supply and demand—women often attack other women if they look or act differently. Shane and I like to think that every woman has various facets to her personality, and she changes and grows through the years. An honest woman makes mistakes. We have, undoubtedly, made mistakes. We are not proud of, unwittingly, being part of an unhealthy beauty message. Yet, we've learned a lot from our experiences.

Women's groups have attacked us when it was obvious that we were victims, too. We understand why that was so easy to do—we were an easy mark. But now more than ever, women need powerful role models in the long run, females who achieve, contribute and succeed in science, business, art, sports, etc. A woman's body is beautiful. But there is not just one type of beauty. Nor should beauty be the sole purpose behind a person's rise to fame.

Women must start blazing their own trails. We live in a bountiful, free country—one of the most sophisticated, wealthy nations in the world—and we have never had a female president. Name 10 U.S. women known for significant political and scientific contributions. Did you stop at number six or seven? And yet, how many of us know what Gwyneth Paltrow wore to last year's Academy awards? Oh, yes, we are, indeed, fortunate to be American women and live in this land of fickle plenty.

As the ultimate consumers, women weave their own web of delusion. We often see fame, success and money as the long-term goal—especially in this town. Playboy's Hugh Hefner once said, "To be successful, you have to be the first of your kind." We think that women's magazines are often far sexier and more titillating than men's publications. And women's magazines outsell men's publications by a long shot. It all comes back to this: female power rests in the women's market. We cannot hope to fight fire with fire in the men's market. Instead, women must choose to put out the fire with a cool stream of education, logical choices and mutual support.

We also do not believe in attacking the media, fashion designers or talent. We should appreciate fashion like we do museum pieces. Do we have to <u>be</u> it to appreciate it? Just because we see a beautiful flower in the field, does not mean we have to pick it. I think some fashion looks great on those gaunt models. Women need to learn to respect a variety of beauty and try not to control it, dictate it, or make one type excessively important. Freedom! Isn't that what feminism is all about?

We—through sheer and utter panic—abused our bodies with extreme diets, laxatives, binges, purges and excessive exercise. Naturally, we felt the pressure to be thin. Destructive, insecure behavioral patterns are usually deep-seated. There's a theory in psychology which says that most women who lean towards stripping, modeling or posing for centerfolds have had absent fathers. Interesting. Maybe early on we did crave "paternal approval," from the world in general, especially since we felt rejected, invisible and abandoned as children and as young women. Bottom line is, we were lucky enough to eventually have role models who supplied the tools for our recovery. And these communication and reasoning tools helped us stop being victims and effect considerable change from within. There are a number of wonderful twelve-step programs available, where women do not persecute, boycott or attack other women.

The word "feminism" has been abused and misconstrued. Feminism, to us, is not about changing women into what other women think they should be. We believe that feminism is supposed to be a support system that affords females the same choices, power, and rights that men have. America has championed women's rights further than most other countries. And yet, the more we battle for equality, the more women obsess about good looks.

By now, you've read this in previous chapters, but it bears repeating: the main issue for compulsive eaters is gaining control of their lives. The pressure of a bad body image is all-consuming, especially if you live in the public eye. Victims often need to "medicate" the mind in order to suppress unwanted feelings. Diets only deal with the symptom (excess weight, flabby things or whatever) and cannot "fix" the underlying emotional problems. Therapy, workshops, support groups and spiritual institutions can help you cope with the underlying problems.

The reason why twelve-step programs are successful is that they treat alcoholism and food disorders as a three-fold disease and focus on a three-fold recovery, which encompasses mental, physical and spiritual solutions. These programs do not put a tiny Band-Aid on a gaping wound. Why not address the reason for the continual mutilation instead of addressing the appearance of the wound?

We have found, through painful trial and error, that the disease usually re-surfaces. Your survival mechanisms may no longer be effective. In your most chronic stages, any addiction is accompanied by feelings of isolation, resignation and unworthiness, as in "no one is as bad as me." We think all obsessive-compulsive diseases are based on dishonesty, denial, self-absorption and unwillingness to surrender. Recovery is based on willingness to surrender and transform your life. From the most personal point of view, we would like to teach you how to eat to live—and not live to eat. That is our goal.

Compulsive Overeaters Anonymous, Anorexia Anonymous and Bulimia Anonymous are just some non-profit support groups. You can find others in your area by looking in your phone book, the local newspaper, library reference, community centers, hospitals or bulletin boards at all self-help centers or bookstores.

List of helpful organizations

American Anorexia/Bulimia Association, Inc.
133 Cedar Lane
Teaneck, New Jersey
(201) 836-1800

ANAD — National Association of Anorexia Nervosa & Associated Disorders
Box 7
Highland Park, IL 60035
(847) 831-3438

ANRED—Anorexia Nervosa & Related Eating Disorders, Inc.
P.O. Box 5102
Eugene, OR 97405
(503) 344-1144

Canopy Cove
Tallahassee, FL
(800) 236-7524

Center for Change
1790 N. State Street
Orem, UT 84057
(801) 224-8255

Green Mountain at Fox Run
Fox Lane, Box 164
Ludlow, VT 05149
(802) 228-8885

Institute of Living
400 Washington Street
Hartford, CT 06106
(800) 673-2411

Hazelden
Has 12 step programs and rehabs for patients 18 years and older for food disorders with drug dependency as primary addiction, as well as recovery programs for other problems.
(800) 257-7800

Laureate Psychiatric
Tulsa, OK
(800) 822-5173

Medical Center at Princeton
Princeton, NJ
(609) 497-4490

Medical University of South Carolina
Charleston, SC
(843) 792-1414
(800) 424-MUSC

The Menninger Clinic
P.O. Box 829
Topeka, KS 66601-0829
(800) 351-9058

Monte Nido
Malibu, CA 90265
(310) 457-9958

The National Anorexia Aid Society
5796 Karl Road
Columbus, Ohio 43029
(614) 436-1112

Overeaters Anonymous, World Service
Rio Rancho, New Mexico
(505) 891-2664

Rader Programs (Inpatient facilities)
Corporate Headquarters
Los Angeles, CA
(800) 841-1515

Remuda Ranch
One East Apache
Wickenburg, AZ 85390
(800) 445-1900

The Renfrew Center
Philadelphia, South Florida, New York and New Jersey
(800) RENFREW

Rogers Memorial Hospital
4700 Valley Road
Oconomowoc, WI 53066
(800) 767-4411

Rosewood
Wickenburg, AZ
(800) 280-1212 or
(877) 74WOMEN
St. Joseph's Hospital
7620 York Road
Baltimore, MD 21204
(410) 427-2100

Shades of Hope
P.O. Box 639
Buffalo Gap, TX 79508
(800) 588-HOPE

Sierra Tucson   *(Inpatient)*
165 N. Lago del Oro Parkway
Tucson, Arizona 85739
(800) 842-4487

Swedish Medical Center
Seattle, WA
(206) 781-6345

Tulane Behavioral Health Center
1040 Calhoun St.
New Orleans, LA 70018
(800) 548-4183

The Willough at Naples
9001 Tamiami Trail East
Naples, FL
(800) 722-0100
(941) 774-4500

For a free mail order catalog of books on eating disorders, send your request for "Eating Disorders Bookshelf Catalog — MPF" to:
Gurze Books
P.O. Box 2238
Carlsbad, CA 92008.
(800) 756-7533

Also:
Health Communications, Inc.
Enterprise Center
3201 S.W. 15th St.
Deerfield, Beach, Florida 33442
(800)851-9100

Scary diet story 17

Holidays and large family celebrations were always exceedingly stressful. They became gatherings of addicts, co-addicts, enablers, (or even "normies"). There were also loved ones and friends who came together to gossip, catch up and indulge in ... FOOD! Now, mind you, we are the feast-or-famine types of dieters. Our motto was to live like saints, eating only communion wafers, with an occasional orgasmic binge to break the rigid dietary rules.

If we planned to use holidays for "reward" binges, then we would have to diet down for the main event. Consider that twisted line of reasoning: A holiday binge is the perfect incentive to starve! When a Christmas or a birthday got really close (let's not even discuss Thanksgiving—you wouldn't believe what happened, anyway), we would radically diet in order to justify our planned binge. If a holiday was weeks away, there would be plenty of time to starve for the occasion and to plan our Roman feasts. The problem was that our diet programs were too strict to continue for weeks on end, and we usually ended up breaking our diet promises and following the urge of the pre-event binge. After this sort of diet miscalculation, we'd always exercise, completely out of control, for the next few weeks.

Some of our finest examples include taste-testing dozens of bags of Halloween candy to ensure that they did not contain poison or razor blades. Easter egg hunting was an art form that demanded practice with chocolate eggs, which regrettably melted with regularity. (That meant replacing those chocolate eggs over and over again before Easter.) You know how much energy it takes to shop for Christmas gifts? One cannot starve when determining what to get for picky relatives. You have to "snack" here and there. And these snacks were often pounds of holiday cookies and entire pecan and pumpkin pies... all to convey the Christmas spirit, naturally. Then, there was something that only came once a year—eggnog! We would start stocking up on eggnog in October—what if stores ran out of our favorite brand on Christmas eve? Horrors!

July Fourth's hot dogs and hamburger bonanzas made us feel very patriotic, and, thus, it was extremely important to devour them prior, in preparation, to the actual occasion. And, please, mark the following note of etiquette: it is terribly rude not to sample a birthday cake before giving it to your special birthday guest. People pleasers? Maybe. But holidays were our favorite excuses for breaking our commitments. We were always utterly miserable when the holiday treats were finally passed around the table—and no sense of anticipation ever remained. Bummer!

Scary diet story 18

While we were on an assignment in Europe, we stayed at one of the most hedonistically luxurious hotels (all expenses paid, as usual). The Louve? The Left Bank? The only sights we wanted to see were the crepe stands and the finer pastry shops.

There was always one day after our photo shoots that we reserved for rest before returning home. That day was actually designated as our "restful" bingeing and purging day. This time, we awoke as usual and started ordering "good" food—meat, cheese, fruit and vegetables. Oh, but how could we leave Paris without tasting their famous baguettes? That would be a crime. And the steak fries and hot buns and berry jellies…

We kept ordering and re-ordering room service from a sweet Frenchman who didn't speak a word of English. He chuckled and shook his head unbelievingly each time we pointed to the next entrée, dessert or snack from the menu. He gladly cleared each empty tray to make room for the next.

The hotel bill told the whole story at check-out. Our expense tab for the first two weeks was close to zero, but on the <u>last</u> day we closed the kitchen and practically *bought* the dining room. Smart employers should have put a limit on our spending that last day.

Chapter 10

𝓜otivational techniques: transformation

The old saying goes, "There are three ways to conceptualize yourself: the way you see yourself; the way others see you, and the way you *really* are. We divide personalities into four groups: (1) "mountains," (2) "people who move mountains," (3) "dirt on the mountains," (4) and "sliders" (people who slide away from the mountains).

"Mountains" are people who are usually famous, wealthy or damn lucky. They allow all of life's perks to come to them, or they let others hustle for them. They are good business people and intelligent visionaries. Many were born into power and riches, or fame fell smack into their lap.

"People who move mountains" are the hustlers; they make things happen. Mountain-movers are self-made successes who are never satisfied; they continually blaze their own paths and reinvent themselves. They usually use money and power as rewards or by-products—money is not their first priority. Movers are constructive and capable of profound wisdom.

Then there are "the dirt on the mountain" types. They are complacent couch potatoes or coattail riders. They're never fulfilled or totally satisfied, but they lack the desire to build or to create on their own. They have no problem living off other people's wealth or success or being a "second banana." They are unmotivated; can be deceitful, and would rather gossip enviously instead of competing. They often give up, but make it look as though they surrender or take a vow of simplicity or poverty by choice. Their motives are unclear, but the goal is often money and power—at any cost. "Dirt-on-the-mountain" types will "sell you out" if the price is right.

Last, there are "sliders," the people who slip away from the "mountains." Have you ever known a person who had glorious opportunities or who was gifted with immense talent, but consistently made bad choices or took reckless actions? This type of person is usually a practicing addict. "The grass is greener on the other side" or "the glass is half empty" typifies the sliders' belief system. "Sliders" never know a good thing until it hits them in the kisser, and then they run from all responsibility. "Sliders" live with unremitting risks by exhibiting reckless behavior, whereas a healthy mountain mover will take healthy risks to open doors to where no man has gone before.

"Sliders" lie, cheat and steal, regularly—just to lie, cheat and steal. They get high on scheming and conning everyone, and they never know what "bottoming out" is, even when they hit it because they are so busy trying to con their way out of a crisis or tragedy. You cannot help them because they don't want your help, and, worse, they'll help you "slide down" with them. They will use all their energies to scheme for a shady motive; yet, it would have been easier and less time-consuming just to get an honest job. If they won the lottery, "sliders" would not have enough money to buy themselves out of the destruction and chaos they have caused.

None of us falls into just one of these purely theoretical models in all aspects of our lives. We can either jump from one category to the other, or we manifest a combination of several categories simultaneously. Maybe we are "mountains" in our career, but "sliders" in our relationships. Yet, we are not condemned to a certain personality or future. We don't like using the word "karma" because it is often misconstrued. However, karma, in any sense of the word, is not fate. We can choose our paths; there ARE choices. Karma is a reaction or the by-product of our choices. Once we make our choice and do the footwork; then the outcome (or karma) is left to God or our Higher Power. We have to take responsibility for the outcome because we make the choices.

That is why recovery is more than just abstaining; recovery means taking responsibility for good choices and their outcome and making amends for past poor choices. How can we ever learn what a good choice is, or what success signifies, unless we learn what defines healthy thinking. Healthy thinking is a good recovery; it is based on rigorous honesty. As they say, it is not easy, but it is simple: truth, courage and acceptance. Our rightful path to health and fitness may not be easy to attain, but it sure makes life easier.

There're not too many people who are naturally enthusiastic about diets and exercise, like some exercise icons. So we try to motivate ourselves so as to help ourselves get to our goal weight, size or shape.

Here are 10 common inspirations:

1. Tune into TV Programs and Fitness Videos.

You can buy or rent exercise videotapes, regardless of your fitness level. Some of the strongest, sexiest women in the fitness industry produce quality exercise aids. Also, various national and cable television program offer effective workouts throughout the day.

2. Prepare Before and After Photos.

Lots of young girls cut out pictures from magazines, of actresses and models they idolize, and paste them on a refrigerator or in a scrapbook. We do not recommend this. Young women comparing themselves to unrealistic, potentially unhealthy role models is a dangerous territory. Instead, we suggest urging your young charge to take her own photograph now and write *"Before"* above it. Then put a label saying, *"After,"* next to the *Before* picture. This is where she will place a future success picture. Maybe you can envision different stages of evolution: *Before, During, Almost Finished, Healthy and Goal Weight*, for example.

3. Build a Buddy System.

This is an instant co-inspiration system. Just make sure that your buddy is as dedicated as you are, and that your fitness and diet levels complement each other. If your buddy flakes out, research shows, it might even be harder for you to stick it out. Choose wisely, and remember: dogs are the most loyal exercise companions!

4. Let Music Move You.

It is proven that music helps the release of motivating brain chemicals—endorphins and serotonin—to make a workout easier. Whether it's Beethoven or the Spice Girls that rock your boat, studies show that listening to music encourages more enjoyable workouts of longer duration.

5. Re-route Your Reward System.

Do not reward a successful diet and exercise goal with food. Train yourself to enjoy other healthy rewards, such as books, movies, shopping or other entertainment. As a reward, we, personally, choose focus on remembering the difference between a binge hangover and a delightfully peaceful sleep after a hard workout. Our best reward during recovery was acknowledging that we'd experienced yet another binge-free day.

6. Keep a Diet and Exercise Journal.

This is so important: Most compulsive overeaters are in denial about their actual food intake and tend to suppress feelings and motives, which will cause them to overeat later. Turn to writing rather than eating. Notice and note your daily improvement—mentally, spiritually, as well as physically.

7. Buy Fabulous Sneakers and Activewear.
Shoes make all the difference. There are some very expensive fitness shoes that make you feel like you're walking on clouds, and there are less expensive shoes that make you feel almost the same way. Nonetheless, cheap shoes may cause chronic foot problems in the future. Always try shoes on before buying and ask an educated salesperson about your prospects. Comfortable, flattering clothes also make a huge difference in your workout attitude; looking good can make you train harder. We think it's best to buy name brands on sale, rather than generic copycats.

8. Read Success Stories.
All health and fitness publications contain amazingly inspiring stories of success. Men's muscle magazines are also chock-full of motivational tips and tales. Occasionally, exchange a basic diet story for one of life inspiration; try a bio on Mother Teresa or Martin Luther King. Reading about one of history's great saints or contributors to Humankind can make your own exercise dilemmas feel like kindergarten playtime.

9. Explore Your Mind with Meditation.
Many theories prove that various meditation techniques help clear the mind, improve memory, decrease stress and lower your blood pressure. Meditation means focus and increased feelings of self-esteem; daily meditation is good medicine.

10. Repeat Mantras and Affirmations.
If you think you can do it, then you can. We know you can do it. Your body does not recognize negativity. If you chant, for example, "I will not eat," your mind is only acknowledging, "I eat." (It does not hear "will not".) It is better to affirm, "I will abstain;" "I am healthy, strong and energetic;" "Happiness and discipline will fill me up and satisfy me." If you are constantly affirming "I hate exercise," you'll figure out a way to avoid it!

How to attain success

We are often asked this common question, in as far as it relates to dieting, recovery or even Hollywood: "How do you attain success?" People make millions selling inspirational tapes or spending bundles gambling on the "luck" of success. Success does not often equate with good luck, however, and there IS no such thing as *continuous* good luck.

If you are persistent—even at roulette—you can make those atoms of energy flow effectively, and you can beat the even toughest odds.

It all comes down to what we call our Triple Ds: Desire, Discipline and Drive. Without desire, the lotto ticket will not be bought; the grand opportunity will be overlooked, and the diet will not begin. Desire is the essence of hope. No one can develop desire for you, however; you must cultivate it on your own. The stronger your desire, the easier the work.

Next is discipline: when you know your goals, you put desire into action—discipline! You write down what it will take to attain success, and which short- and long-term actions you must take in order to manifest your goals. But, be careful what you wish for and try to match your desires to your needs. Unless you are too disordered to make short-term goals, do not let others dictate them to you. (In this case, only qualified specialists or sponsors should teach discipline.) It helps to choose a wise role model and then simulate their method of discipline. Your discipline, in recovery, may be as easy as surrendering to a therapist and/ or sponsor. But only you can do that footwork.

Finally, drive is the energy that keeps you going in the dark night of the soul. This is usually when most people give up, whether it's rejection from a job or exhaustion during a marathon. Losers look for a new high or honeymoon when the going gets tough or boring. You are not a loser as long as you do not give up! A lot of people ask, "What if I fail?" Our answer is, "I'm so busy getting back up and do not have time to acknowledge defeat! I will die <u>trying</u>!" It is persistence and consistency that matters the most. It is better to have a 15-minute steadfast workout every day, than to overdo and burn out.

Each of the triple D's can't exist without the other two. They work synergistically, not magically. I always made fun of people spending millions on "good luck" or spending precious time finding shortcuts. Just get out there and do it, but do it right. Hey, if <u>we</u> can do it—no joke—you can do it, too!

This quote is from Ken Wahl: "The definition of success is relative. For me, it is peace and simplicity. Ambition is fine, as long as it does not take you over. Then it is obsession."

Scary diet story 19

We love horses more than anything. One of our original purposes for modeling was to finance our expensive horse hobby. So, one of our most exciting offers, in our heyday, came from R.D. Hubbard, owner of the Hollywood Park Racetrack. He wanted to name one of his favorite racehorses "Barbi Twin," and he registered the pretty filly with the Jockey

Association. When we heard this great news, I was suffering with stomach problems related to bulimia and couldn't get too excited.

As life imitates art, within the next few weeks, we heard that *Barbi Twin* had begun compulsively eating, too. In fact, she came down with very bad colic and had to be turned out to pasture. Any chance of racing or showing the horse was quickly over for Hubbard—though we appreciated the gesture. (In horses, colic is a disease sometimes caused by overeating.) Because horses cannot purge or regurgitate, they bloat, which is very dangerous. Sometimes fatal. So our darling little equine clone turned out to have a food disorder, just like us. But the poor filly tried to binge without purging. Pity, we couldn't teach her some diet tricks...

However, we did share our experience with her—through pure pony prayers. We recently heard a rumor that she had earned a 90-day chip for grain abstinence in HA—Hayaholic Anonymous.

Scary diet story 20

In our pre-laxative days, we relied heavily on over-exercising to shed pounds. Marathons were like religious holidays for us—we've run dozens. It was a challenge to commit to pain and receive more pain—all in the name of fitness. In those days, we had no boundaries or shut-off buttons and could work out until we could not walk. Horrible muscle cramps in the middle of the night provided for very sweet dreams.

To prepare for a book convention at a huge televised event, we were doing our usual six-hour cardio workout. For added incentive to be lean and mean at the promotion, we bought new miniskirts. It felt like our legs were wound with wire on our way to the airport—we'd really overdone it. Our bodies were extremely sore, dehydrated and cramping badly on the plane ride heading toward the event. We weren't looking forward to wearing our hooker high heels for the following evening's events, either.

The next night we were nervous and could barely walk. We wore our familiar cowboy boots on the limo ride over and tried to calm each other's jitters. Just as we were about to strut our stuff down a catwalk across the convention center, we donned our shoes, and I discovered a big problem. My sister—who I pet-named Einstein after this one—had packed for me (not herself, of course)—TWO LEFT HIGH HEELS.

I was already in a sad shape—I felt like a war vet, limping across the stage to receive a medal. Oh, my bulging leg muscles glowed with glory, and yes, I was even complimented for my throbbing, aching thighs. Thanks to my two left shoes, the press photos of that event captured the pain in my face and the bitterness towards my sister. I could have cheerfully killed her.

Chapter 11

Friends, family, co-addicts, enablers and intervention

Here are various definitions that will help you better understand your troubled loved ones. Sometimes, the hardest thing to do is continue to be compassionate, accepting and loving.

Compulsive Overeater

One who eats compulsively. Boy, that gives you an open field to define your own idea of abstinence from obsessive overeating. Abstinence, in recovery, is not a diet plan—it's how the plan is carried out. It implies that the person attempting recovery will eat three planned meals each day with nothing in between. This prevents meal obsession and all-day pig-outs.

For a compulsive eater, certain foods are "triggers" making us go hog-wild. Mine is sugar. So, just like alcoholics do with booze, I steer clear from sugar. I try to avoid it—one day at a time. If I gulp my meal obsessively, trying to relieve stress or fill a void, it eventually triggers a binge. Compulsive eating embodies the feeling of constant hunger, as though nothing you eat is ever enough. There are no shut-off valves. You feel that no one can help, and, thus, hopelessness draws you back to the solution AND your reason for depression—FOOD. But there is hope. Do not let your deeply set dysfunctional behavior overwhelm you. Trust God and allow yourself to surrender to a recovery program. You will see results.

Co-Dependent

There are many definitions, but the simplest is—"someone addicted to the addict." Our definition is also "someone who loses themselves in someone else or other people (people-pleasing)." Co-dependents love to control, fix, rescue and become caretakers. They will brush your hair, fix your breakfast, and drive you anywhere. But this behavior should not be confused with true generosity. Co-dependents make it abundantly clear to everyone that they are the poor, martyred victim who always "give" and get abused. They have a motive: they are addicted to being needed and to complaining about it.

Co-Addict

Co-dependent with the addict. Co-addict is also addicted to the same 'drug of choice,' the addict is addicted to. The co-addicts' dependency is without regard to consequences.

Enabler

An enabler can be a co-dependent, but his or her motive is to make the situation easier for everybody. Enablers refrain from truth, confrontations or uneasy situations. They want to please, look good, suck up, win over and keep peace at any cost. They actually harm the addict because even when they don't encourage the 'drug of choice,' they are silently condoning it if they're not honest and up-front. They may bitch or lecture to the addict, but their actions reinforce the addiction. They may be (or choose to be) in denial. Just their non-confrontational presence alone is a form of denial.

Anorexia

Anorexia Nervosa is an obsessive-compulsive personality disorder, which focuses on the fear of causing weight gain. Research has also found this fear to be a psychological reason not to eat. Anorexics live in a constant state of extreme stress and anxiety. This is due to the high levels of serotonin, which are made by overactive neurotransmitters in the hypothalamus. The anorexic feels a loss of control, and therefore feels the need to take control by eating less or no food (often 1000 calories fewer). Tryptophane, which is found in a lot of foods, is a precursor of serotonin. This is why an anorexic instinctively feels the need to avoid food, in order to keep the serotonin levels down. This constant "fight or flight" state causes extra cortical and adrenal hormones to be manufactured which, in turn, interrupts APV — a hormone responsible for appetite. That lack of APV distinguishes anorexics from bulimics.

Bulimia

Bulimics have the same obsessive compulsive personality disorder and control issues with perfection, food and weight as do anorexics, but after depriving their bodies of food, bulimics break their fast with large masses of food (this process is called bingeing). This happens because bulimics, (as opposed to anorexics) haven't had the APV destroyed. The over-accumulated APV causes a tremendous appetite. This cycle effects a pattern of highs and lows, making bulimics seem erratic in behavior. After a binge, it is common for a bulimic to purge and/or obsessively exercise for hours. Recognizing the problem is half the battle.

Both anorexia and bulimia diseases are grounded in denial. Balanced wholesome diets can help restore missing chemicals. Professional help and support groups are a must. Stress management control and APV shots have been recommended for anorexics. One of the first things both anorexics and bulimic need to know in order to get well, is that they are not in control. When such surrender process begins, the afflicted will elevate to a higher level of faith and hope.

Adult Children of Alcoholics (ACA)

My definition of an ACA is simple: they are victims of parents or caretakers who are addicts of some kind. ACA (including Shane and me) have three tremendous disadvantages: genetic inheritance of the disease, learned behavior, and shame (feeling responsible). ACA learn to hide, steal, lie and cheat for or because of the addicts' disease. This set of patterns is the distinction of the disease. It completely destroys their life and distorts their thinking, just like that of the addict or abuser). But as adults, we can choose not to continue being victims, we can stop the blaming and forgive our parents (or caretakers) for being sick. There are many successful people who are recovered addicts or adult children of addicts. Much of their success can be attributed to a hard-core, rigorously honest recovery program.

Body Dysmorphic Disorder

Today, BDD is a growing phenomenon: The main symptoms are body-obsession and a distorted perception of physical imperfections. Studies have shown that BDD victims may have a chemical brain imbalance, including very low levels of serotonin. BDD victims obsess to the point of over-correcting their "flaw" by excessive exercise, hardcore dieting, or even total isolation. It takes over their life, akin to many health and dieting dysfunctions.

All of the above-mentioned disorders have this in common: control and perfectionism (or the lack of it) along with fear and shame. That's why, if recovery focuses merely on a food and nutrition plans, eating or not eating, and not on the underlying psychological issues, the physical manifestations of the disorder will reappear. Only a full-fledged recovery program can turn the tide.

Having a twin, I can say it is worse to see a loved one destroy herself with a self-inflicted disease, rather than experience it yourself. It is a very helpless and powerless feeling. There are many programs (especially 12-Step programs) for alcoholic/drug addicts' family members and loved ones. These programs are good for anyone, because alcohol, like food, is only a symptom. It is the behavior patterns that the programs are effective with.

There are also numerous new programs and literature for the parents of anorexics and bulimics. Unfortunately, compulsive overeaters have a stigma attached to their sickness, and it's barely considered a disease. Most overeaters are referred to as "weak." Ironically, the heaviest people we've known have endured the strictest food deprivation and dieted to extremes with extraordinary will power. They sacrificed friendships through isolation and self-loathing because they believed they were a mistake. Their survival mechanism (food) filled the void they initially wanted to fill with love. Then food became the biggest issue and the reason for being unloved. This creates a hateful cycle: food at one time was their only ally, the unconditional lover and their single coping method.

Many of us associate food with cozy family gatherings, childhood rewards, or stress relievers. Commercials show thin people eating mounds of crap, and yet heavy people are portrayed as the butt of fat jokes, weak weirdoes or filthy perverts. Such mixed messages we grow up with! Who really knows why we practice destructive behaviors. It is more important to identify them and work on solutions. And as co-addicts, we must educate ourselves instead of trying to "fix" the addict. Be available when she reaches out for help. Consuming a box of cookies, alarming weight loss, or constant dieting is a cry for help. But we can actually do more harm than good, if we do not educate ourselves and recognize the difference between denial and enabling.

Compulsive overeating, as with anorexia, bulimia or alcoholism, is a deadly disorder. It is a slow suicide. The destructive behavior will prevail. Not only can an overeater just die from a heart attack or other health crises, she can also regress into severe depression which may lead to desperate actions, or even suicide.

I believe that recovery is impossible without abstinence or sobriety first. Food, purging, or the "drug of choice" may only be the symptoms, but it is absurd trying to penetrate an intoxicated or sick person's wall of defense when they are practicing their disease. Furthermore, if sobriety focuses only on getting "dry" without a psychological recovery, then the sobriety is usually temporary. A recovery program is based on a system of solutions with black and white choices of actions. The rigid pattern helps the addict mentally, physically and spiritually. There are many different programs or recovery paths to take.

I think that a big mistake co-addicts or outsiders often make is that they address the symptom as the only problem and/or cure. If an anorexic gains weight, they think they are well. Not true. When people used to alarmingly tell me I was scarily thin, I'd say, "Thank you!" Yet, on the other hand, when I was heavier, and someone remarked on my rear, "Wow, baby has back," it would trigger me to head for the nearest donut shop.

For a compulsive overeater, there is nothing worse than a food cop. We will find ways to manipulate, seduce, blackmail, barter, "closet eat," or threaten for ways to practice our disease. To have outside circumstances as the foundation for our willpower (a controlled environment) can be dangerous. If there is a "slip" or an opening to take your own action, your willpower will be gone! We're usually obsessed with finding ways to circumvent rigid rules and to open locked cabinets.

Yet, I do believe in "rehabs" for "drying out". Only because we are creatures of habit and if a habit is "enforced" (and grooved in the brain) as we detox, we are more susceptible to sobriety. But rehabs, institutions or "controlled environments" seem to only work when therapy is incorporated. And this can't come from loved ones or family members, as they are usually too co-dependent and controlling. Moreover, these disorders usually affect the whole family. Powerful abstinence environment and the presence of well-qualified specialists, as well as the presence of other recovering addicts in group therapy—encompass the factors of successful recovery.

The disease starts "setting in" when a major self-absorption surfaces its ugly head. So to try to force the anorexic, for example, to eat and not to lose weight is going in the wrong direction. I think it is like telling a druggy to use a clean needle instead of a dirty one. The disease is still there, always will be, and can come back to exactly where it was, or worse. It can also be transmitted from one deadly form to another or from one person to another. So many people morphed their disorder into an obsession with the person they fell in love with. They may have lost their eating disorder, but they also lost their identity. Some even end up in worse depression and suicide, as well. Same problems and issues—just a different disease with a different symptom.

One of the saddest mistakes I've witnessed is what some mothers do with their anorexic daughters. They become obsessed with their daughter's weight loss and the loss of control over her. All the while the daughter drifts further out of touch and loses ever-more weight. This mother-daughter battle only keeps the energy and focus on the daughter's body, which will be never good enough for someone in full-blown disease. I'm not saying denial is the answer. Of course, dramatic weight loss is alarming, and friends and family should be concerned. However, learn how to help before you intervene.

Intervention is a tough, usually misconstrued subject. My sis and I have been through interventions, participated in interventions and even avoided interventions. Please, note the difference between intervening and meddling. Intervention should be done objectively and should concentrate on the issue, not attack the person. Remember, she already feels shame and victimization; shaming her further will not help. Give the sick person the chance to come clean without condemning or condoning her behavior.

Meddling

This is dealing with the ego and opinion, not focusing on facts. Meddling is condescending and is a form of control (i.e., being co-dependent). You can place your own boundaries, limits and rules, but threats, blackmail or bribes <u>do not work</u>. Remember: Your loved one is not bad or wrong, she is sick!

The expression "in secrets lies sickness" holds very true. Intervention, by definition, is "to come, appear, or lie between two things." Intervention worked for us when sober loved ones did not lecture. This disease affects everyone in the family.

The other extreme is "tough love," full of lectures and reprimands. This always makes the addict more fearful and forces the regression back into isolation. Anorexics and bulimics create rigid rituals in order to control their boundaries and environment.

If, in recovery, food addicts learn to cultivate other interests, their obsessions will lessen. Eating disorder victims are often overly self-absorbed, so charity and contribution are part of the paths to recovery. Why? It takes the ego—"me"—syndrome out of the daily routine. When recovering addicts help others, they should also be aware of the harm they may unintentionally inflict on others. We are sick, deluded and confused. By alerting our loved ones, gently, we can learn to become responsible for our own and their recovery and stop hurting the people we love the most.

Let's summarize: intervention should be conducted with a specialist in a safe, loving environment.

- Help your loved one let go of her secret; she is no longer fooling anyone but herself. Let her know that a food disorder is a progressive disease, and that everyone knows about her problem.

- Make her feel safe enough to open up, cry, let feelings surface, and encourage discussion when she is depressed or isolated.

- As a family, get involved with other things, which change the energy from body obsession to healthy pursuits. Giving an addict a monetary reward or encouraging her to model, or even giving her a new dress, is not a good idea. Make her see how you recognize the seriousness of the sickness.   But give hope and support her in recovery.

- Recovery: You have no control over someone who is truly sick. You can set the example and rules to follow, for recovery, but you cannot enforce them. Sometimes all you can do is just NOT enable. Do not lecture, but don't pretend that there is no problem or that you are not affected by it. You can also attend group therapy where other parents, relatives, friends and partners are likewise affected by their loved ones. Surrendering your obsession does not mean surrendering concern; it means surrendering control.

Enabling

This is often misunderstood. People think, for example, that enabling is just pouring alcohol for an alcoholic. The "trickiest" enablers are the co-dependents. They are the poor, innocent martyrs who try to "rescue" or "cure" the addict. They appear as though they are helping the addict get well because they will bitch, sacrifice, beg and lecture. A very sick addict can become progressively sicker, with a good enabler.

Denial

Defined as a refusal to comply with or satisfy a request, or to grant the truth (contradiction). Enabling can appear as helpfulness, whereas denial is simply refusal to address the addiction or aid recovery. Denial is a form of enabling; if you refuse to admit the disease, then you actually condone the disease. Addicts are already in denial about addiction and the seriousness of it, so your denial reinforces the pretense that their secret is safe.

Maybe, you will find it impossible to be honest with the addict. This doesn't mean you also have to be in denial. People respect honesty. It represents courage and strength, which, ironically, the addict searches for in her own addiction. You have no power over her, but you can set a strong example by not living in denial yourself.

We all use denial to suppress pain or uncomfortable feelings. Confrontation is something we all try to refrain from; it is our nature to be agreeable and pleasing. So instead of diplomatically confronting the addict, co-addicts will sometimes suppress the truth until they explode at an inappropriate time. The first action is admitting to the disease and being honest with its influence. That is the beginning of finding solutions.

Relapse

This phenomenon is defined as returning to a former state of illness; it may occur unexplainably and unexpectedly. One can be on a long-term, hard-core recovery path, and, suddenly, with no explanation, relapse occurs. This return to your addictive behavior usually means that you'll go back to where you left off, or worse. Interestingly, the memory of the disease stays intact.

Addiction can creep up in the most subtle, sneaky ways, especially if you are in denial. Brain chemistry has natural "regulators," and overindulgence helps deplete these chemicals, so your "shut off" buttons don't work. Most people go through a "dry out" or natural "rehab" session on their own. All bodies have that capability. But it's tricky because—without warning—the body's regulators may shut down completely, and willpower is useless against that.

Let me reiterate that addiction is not just a physical disease. Stopping the "symptoms," such as over-eating, purging, etc., is necessary, but not sufficient. You need to change the brain patterns, which encompass your "life style" and "attitude." Those are the mental and spiritual ingredients of the disease and recovery. You have to cultivate healthy replacement behaviors. As I've said before, you have to "put deposits in the bank for your emergency withdrawals when needed." A "slip" is when you return to your addiction in a subtle form. It may seem "innocent," but therein lies a warning that you are returning to old behavioral patterns which will take you back, will cause you to crave "old ways" to "deal" or "escape."

When someone reminisces about the "good ol' days" and envies a "normal" person who does not need to abstain from their addiction, that thinking is equivalent to heading for a slip. Recovery is based on the <u>actions</u> of honesty, amends and gratefulness. "White-knuckling", dry drunks or controlled environments (in contrast to programs of responsible discipline) all wind up causing "slips" or a full-blown relapse. There's a saying that once you're back to practicing your addiction, the "high" might not be as good as it was, but getting back on the road to recovery is much harder and more humiliating. So do not set yourself up by testing yourself (putting the fawn in front of the lion), kidding yourself (denial) or getting too tired, too lonely, too hungry, or too angry.

Relapse can be a good learning experience. It will teach you that the disease is always waiting to surface — without you daily examining your motives, attitudes and priorities. Of course, it is likely that you will slip. There is no such thing as a "cure" or being "born again," in recovery. You do not have to affirm you're sick. Just do not deny it. But you do have to affirm that your sickness can take over you at any time if you are in denial and do not follow a healthy recovery program.

One should not live in fear of relapse, however. We should be cautious and humble and remember that addiction almost killed us and distorted our mental capability. Living one day at a time, doing the footwork, will take us that much farther from our addiction and closer to a sane and serene life. It is important that one should get outside help (perhaps, in spiritual programs), rather than rely on isolation or willpower. Your mind is incapable of healthy and sane thoughts when you are sick. Remember, the disease takes your brain hostage when you're practicing your drug of choice or are not in full recovery. As long as you realize that, you are halfway down the road of recovery.

The other part of recovery is to work on solutions in the context of very regimented black and white actions. I think that 90% of the problem in these diseases is the "control" issue and trying to rely on our own willpower. When we surrender to qualified specialists, group therapy with other addicts and/or a Higher Power, we are letting go of control. We are obviously out of control when we're in our disease state. We think we are "weak" or do not have discipline and willpower, if we "surrender". On the contrary. It takes strength and courage to "let go" of habits and rituals that may not work but make us feel safe. Only God can help us make a needed miracle. But He gives us "tools" (therapy, literature, etc.) to help us do the footwork. God helps those who help themselves.

Scary diet story 21

We could never make any money as movie reviewers—Siskel and Ebert we aren't. Our flick picks totally depended on our moody diet behavior. If we were starving, for instance, we had to watch a movie that was bone-chillingly scary or knee-slappingly funny. A love story was way too corny for us when we hadn't eaten in three days.

But more important than the movie genre, were the meals filmed in the movie! Forget character development, where are the kitchen and restaurant scenes? We had to avoid very sad story lines, too; they might have struck a melancholy chord and triggered a BIG binge. If a brave dog died unexpectedly in a movie, for instance, we'd start devouring anything in sight. On the contrary, if we were in the middle of a binge, we could not stand to watch any blood and guts movies. That would ruin our popcorn digestion. And forget foreign films: we were way too busy passing the junky finger foods back and forth to be able to read subtitles.

Watching movies will always be a diet escape for us. Our movie objective was to supplement the eye entertainment with the mouth entertainment. In one extremely good murder movie a few years back, Shane and I were appalled that the killer (after killing his dog, family and co-workers) left his piece of cake half-eaten and picked up the silly gun. Was he *crazy?*

Scary diet story 22

All flight attendants that have served the Barbi Twins have experienced our radical feast-to-famine binges. We try to nap in order to thwart the airplane-food temptation, but it doesn't always work that way. Once, a zealous flight attendant woke me up *three times* to make sure I didn't want the snack she offered. Of course I wanted the damn cookie! My blood sugar was slumped, the smells from the galley were a sugar-fix crime, and I could practically taste those chips a-melting on my tongue… Didn't she realize that food is a CRIME when you're heading TO a modeling gig?

Flying home on the same airline, we ran into Little Miss Helpful again. Now she was at *our* mercy—we kept her running back and forth for cookies and other edibles during the entire five-hour flight! We didn't mind waddling off the plane bare-foot (our feet were swollen) as long as we could clench cookies in each fist and stuff then down our back pockets for later.

Chapter 12

The road to recovery

We do not intend to break anonymity or "tradition" with our references to Overeaters Anonymous or any other twelve-step program mentioned. Please note that we are not experts in that field, and we do not endorse particular programs. However, we feel it was necessary to share our knowledge and our sense of hope.

We would like to answer three specific questions about recovery that always come up for us:

1. *Are you cured?*
2. *When did you learn that you had a problem, and when did you recover?*
3. *How do you stay thin?*

Well, to start with, we were very lucky to have a therapist mother, who is a recovered twelve-stepper with a lot of experience in recovery. Although, she both educated us and made us aware of our tendencies towards "isms" (intoxicating ourselves with <u>any</u> addictive behavior to suppress feelings), she also let us muddle through our own growth process.

You can exit out of an elevator at any floor—she would tell us—you do not have to hit bottom. Everyone's "bottom" is different, of course. And although we are twins, Shane and I still could not share or choose our respective "bottoms" any more than our mother could. Recovery is an ongoing process with many different faces. As long as you strive for progress and not perfection—and as long as you know mistakes are part of the bargain—then you must continue to learn.

Recovery can start when you identify your character defects so they are not in command of you. It's such a relief to finally realize that recovery means letting go of control and outside circumstances and digging deep down to work on yourself. Maybe you can't change overnight, but you should not let the outside world endanger your peace, progress and goals. The key words are <u>ongoing</u> and <u>attitude</u>. There is no "cure" for alcoholism, bulimia, anorexia, etc. (This answers the first question above.)

Instead of a cure, there is an "ongoing" recovery, which depends on your willingness. And willingness is in your attitude:

- *Are you willing to give up the things that do not work?*
- *Are you willing to commit to a new, healthy path?*
- *Are you willing to be grateful? Grateful does not mean complacent, by the way. Complacent people live in denial and only take what's in front of them because they are unwilling to create new directions.*
- *Are you willing to trust your intuition? Take off your thinking cap and turn to your instincts for what feels right and good. Our minds are crowded with the layers of delusions that we've built to survive our pain. Intuition will help you see new possibilities.*

In our pre-teens, we began to intuitively know that our family life was not "The Waltons." We knew that there were abnormal secrets in our home. No one talked about the alcohol abuse, the presence of religion and the fall or success. The issues themselves were not the real problems, though. The way we dealt with those issues turned into a problem. Put us in the midst of a major crisis, and we would be heroes. Yet if we broke a nail, it could be catastrophic because we were unable to express and communicate our feelings and problems normally. We did not make mistakes; we thought we WERE the mistakes.

Although we saw our mother get recovery at a very early age, we thought that as long as we didn't drink or do drugs, we would not fall victim to addiction. We, however, had addictive personalities which manifested in everything: food and getting rid of it, body obsession, horses, men, co-dependency, agoraphobia, never being good enough (having to be #1), hiding and giving up (even suicidal thoughts) — and not necessarily in that order. We had an empty void as young children, which had nothing to do with our parents. I think that God gives us all this "thirst" so that we could strive for better or different paths and be able to progress and grow. But some of us would rather "avoid" or "mask" these uncomfortable growth experiences with destructive "fixes," to get rid of these unusual feelings.

There were different phases of revelation, epiphany, or just plain recovery that we went through. It is not as though you're just "reborn" with a new, problem-free life. There are different levels. Nothing in life stays the same. It either progresses or regresses. So if you do not continue growing, you'll stagnate or, worse, retreat. It is easy going back to old familiar patterns. After all, we have more experience in that domain. But the good thing is, sobriety is not just about abstaining, it is also about dealing with your life on an honest level instead of focusing on denial, which actually caused the sickness.

Recovery is about making amends, not so much in the form of confessing, but in the context of making sure that we do not repeat our old destructive mistakes.

I remember our mom reminiscing about how we changed at an early age. She said that it broke her heart when she saw the corrupt world influence our innocence. What she saw was my sister and I reacting to the outside world in a "people-pleasing" manner. This was an easy way to be "accepted" or to fit in. We never caved into drugs or alcohol or sexual promiscuity. But she saw us "lose" ourselves in someone else or in trying to be someone else. I think the hardest thing for a parent or loved one to go through is to helplessly watch someone painfully experience life and its disappointments. Our mother did a lot of praying. Thank God, she was not a stage mother. She gave us the freedom to make our own mistakes and to choose the path of recovery.

Even for my sister and I, to see each other go through life's pain, without any influence on each other, was very frustrating. What's worse than seeing someone you love actually fall? Well, it is looking like them, having their reputation, and yet having absolutely no power or control to help them. This is when surrender is important. God helps those who help themselves. "Themselves" is a key word. We can only work on ourselves and set a silent example. I'd rather watch someone jump a horse than have them tell me how to jump the horse. It is more inspiring and motivating that way. And it goes the other way, as well. I'm glad to have seen the pain and mistakes in my family — they helped me have the freedom to make the right choices.

What extremes have my sister and I lived! At one point, we actually tried to join a nunnery, yet we modeled our way to the status of centerfold pin-ups. We lived in places that were nearly slums, to palaces in foreign lands. We've been there, done it. And you know what? We do not regret a thing! I'd rather see the glass half full than half empty. People ask us if we are sorry about our childhood, if we are sorry about our family life (which was more like the Addams Family than the Brady Bunch) or if we are sorry about doing Playboy. That's like asking if I enjoyed having the measles. It was all necessary to get to this point. Maybe it wasn't always enjoyable at the time, but the by-product made us develop empathy, courage, discrimination and vehement commitment. Not many enjoy working out, but in order to get the end result — a well-sculptured muscle— we have to sweat. If not, we'd all be con artists trying to find an easier, softer way. No such thing. This reminds me of a compulsive gambler who believes that he is going to be the one-in-a-billion who outsmarts the odds. Wisdom is not about having to suffer your own lowest "bottoming out;" it is about applying others' experiences and strengths to your own life, so that you no longer have to suffer.

Life itself was therapy for my sister and me because we no longer wanted to be victims or to blame, and we saw a crisis as an opportunity or a challenge to overcome. We experimented with all kinds of religions, therapy, workshops, and even magical "fixes." If I merely participated in one program, such as OA (Overeaters Anonymous), it would have made me think that if I just fixed the food disorder, I would be fine.

However, the food disorder was merely a symptom. I related a great deal to hardcore alcoholics in AA and understood that alcohol was merely their drug of choice. I realized that addiction spans all "isms," and I knew that I didn't have to practice other "isms" to understand them. I realized that addictive disorders stemmed from fear, guilt, shame, dishonesty and resentment.

Many "normies" do not want to label these behaviors as "diseases." They'd rather call a compulsive overeater weak-willed, an alcoholic—a lush, or a bulimic—gross. To me a disease is manifested when some behavioral pattern becomes addictive. This addictive "survival mechanism" that may have worked for some problems, actually becomes the problem. The problem becomes addictive, and the addict is no longer controlled by her will, intelligence or intuition, but by sheer destructive habits, so heavily grooved in the brain that it seems only death can stop them. The addict is dictated by her addiction and will go to any extreme, at any cost (including losing her life), to practice it. I've yet to see someone actually enjoy her addiction in its later stage. Of course, I've witnessed practicing alcoholics, whose disease tolerated their adhering to a two-faced double life. They look normal and functional when it is necessary, and only get drunk and out-of-control, when it is "appropriate." But the disease is powerful and sneaky, and with a cloak of denial that seems to nourish it. I'm not qualified, nor do I have an interest in "outing" other people's "ism." I just know from our experience that the disease is powerful, and the recovery is freedom.

It is ironic how most people fall into addictions searching for the feeling of freedom, so that they can refrain from rigid rules, religious no-nos, or even man's laws. Addiction is your worst prison. Recovery trains one to find relief and freedom in discipline or discrimination. Who wants to be dictated by every whim, desire, thirst or request? We learned in recovery to put our needs and desires on the playing field. Recovery is not about deprivation, but on the contrary, it is about being able to allow ourselves to live at our fullest and best, which our addictions do not permit us to do at all.

We did—and still do—all forms of recovery. Daily meditation, twelve steps, literature, church, contribution, amends, commitments, and shar-ing our experience, strength and hope. We know we still have a long way to go, but we're enjoying the process, rather than waiting for the "visions and fireworks" at the end of the rainbow.

Oh, and about staying thin, it is the same thing. Our obsession made us overweight, anorexic, etc. As long as you're in recovery and not eat-ing over issues (with the right committed daily diet and fitness program), you will "level out" to what you're supposed to be. As I said before, you do the footwork, and let God take care of the results. But best of all, we're grateful. We could not have survived without the "gifts" of our wonderful, spiritual family, especially our parents, aunt and uncle. Our lives have been full of opportunities and sharing, and we count our bless-ings every day.

If I were to put it in a nutshell, life is a paradox. Things or symbols we use to express our freedom (even from extremely rigid rules and disci-pline) become an addiction, which puts us in a much more rigid prison. So, obliterating these addictions, with some discipline and God's help, relieves us to actually experience true freedom.

I think that the trick to recovery is to replace addiction with a healthy lifestyle. Otherwise, you're white-knuckling it or you are a "dry drunk." For example, instead of turning to diets, donuts or drugs to escape sup-pressed feelings, find a way of expressing them so that they do not mani-fest in a destructive behavior that usually turns into an addiction. Writ-ing, group therapy, or somehow "investing" in your self-worth can cre-ate a transformation. The problem will always be there — if you do not confront it. So will the addiction. Just make the replacement more entic-ing or more of a habit. Pretty soon the addiction will be just a memory. But it should be a memory, which we never forget. We must remember that addiction could surface again if we do not spot-check our "inven-tory." Do not invest in another person — invest in your own spiritual growth — it means you're investing in yourself, as well as others. This makes you whole. Spiritualism, to my sister and me, is an awareness of our "gifts" and how to use them to benefit both others and ourselves. That coincides with sobriety … what a coincidence!

Really, I think my disease is a "blessing in disguise." If my recovery only allowed me to have a perfect body, how could I progress mentally or spiritually? Literally, in order to stay "sober," one has to "clean up" all aspects of one's life and behavior. When Shane and I cleaned up our diet, we didn't just manifest good bodies; we also attained a top fitness level, good health and clear thinking. What's the use of looking good if the obsession is still there, preventing us from enjoying feeling good?

Scary diet story 23

What does a bulimic/anorexic dread the most? We call it The Twilight Zone BLOAT! Sometimes it creeps up in the middle of the night, like the bogeyman. Who knows if it was hormones, too much salt in the frozen dinner, or hidden fat in the frozen yogurt made by unscrupulous yogurt manufacturers? Bloat is the bulimic's regular morning hangover, and all you know is that your body's mysteriously expanding like a helium balloon.

When your eyes are slits, and your rings don't cover your knuckles, be smart enough to stay away from the mirror. When this happened during the disease years, I'd quickly cancel all my "unimportant" meetings: work, a doctor's appointment, and even a date. The only appointment I was concerned with was the one at the gym.

Then, God forbid, don't let the phone ring or a neighbor stop to chat while I'm on my way to the health club. The frenzy starts the second I turn the ignition. I proceed to give a whole new meaning to "flipping the bird" to other drivers... outta my way!

One day just a few years ago, I got a flat tire while hysterically trying to get to the gym. It was in the middle of a local road, at the bottom of a hill in a remote area. I screamed in frustration and had a full-blown tantrum. Finally, I waved a few cars over to help me. But, I didn't have time to waste helping them do their good deed. I told them I had to make a phone call because I was late, and they could continue while I jogged up the hill. I felt so devilishly guilty getting my way while I had these suckers take care of my responsibilities!

Five hours later, I ran back down the hill ... my car was stolen! Oh, I knew I brought on the bad karma. I went to a call box and phoned the police who explained that my car had merely been towed. They asked what I had been doing for the last few hours, and I told them I'd forgotten my Prozac that morning. I told them that if I hadn't jogged for the last five hours, I'd have become suicidal. Surprisingly, they understood (it wasn't too far from the truth, after all). They drove me to the impound yard, while I sat in the back of the police car, grinning from ear-to-ear.

Scary diet story 24

The favorite question of the week posed to Hal, our frazzled family pharmacist, was: "What can we do to lose thirty pounds in ten days without getting weak?" Mind you, this man is not your average corner pharmacist. Hal has the skills of a Nobel Prize scientist; he knows every trick, diet, drug and supplement. This is why, quickly initiated, he became an immediate family member.

Hal was actually an anti-drug and pro-vitamin proponent and would annoyingly mouth these depressing words: "Moderation, balance and slow weight loss are the only ways to go." But we also knew how to "work him," so that he'd tell us about the new secret diet that top stars were using. Hal would regularly warn us, "This could make you very sick," or "It will only be temporary weight loss." Or even, "It is dangerous, don't try it."

His paternal concern often did guide us in the right direction. He saw us fail at every diet known to mankind. He saw us at every dress size and never showed surprise. It got to the point that when we called him, he would no longer ask, "How are you?" He would ask, "What diet are you on now?" Hal had it rough with the Barbi Twins for years.

Today, it's so pleasant (isn't it Hal?) to call him up to discuss family crises, the weather, anything at all, except diets. He is a great therapist, too. We think that Hal has lost a lot of weight worrying about our deadly nutritional habits, so he had to retire early just to get away from our furious interrogations. Hal's big mistake was giving us his home number so we could also befriend his wonderful family. But that's another story.

Scary diet story 25

All-you-can-eat "mono" diets were our favorites: pick one nutritious staple and eat just that for seven days. One busy summer, our pick-of-the-week was watermelons because they're sweet, filling and huge! We'd stuff ourselves until we couldn't bend over. And, naturally, we wouldn't venture out of the house because we were constantly urinating like racehorses.

Weighing in on the sixth morning, we scratched our heads in consternation because we hadn't lost an ounce. True, we were each consuming the equivalent of six large watermelons a day, but that's all we ate. We rationalized that we needed an "anti-cleansing" diet, and sat down to a gargantuan breakfast at our favorite diner: French toast, pancakes, bagels, muffins, hash browns and hot chocolate. When the waitress asked if we also wanted a side dish of fruit, Shane and I gestured hysterically with our hands (our mouths were stuffed), "No way!"

Chapter 13

Most frequently asked questions ... and answers

Nutrition, diet and exercise

Q *Which diet worked for you and which failed?*

A All of them worked, and then all of them failed. They all worked at first, and then they stopped working. That's what always happens when you restrict calories and deprive yourself of a healthy, balanced lifestyle.

Q *How do you get enough exercise without over-exercising?*

A We set strict limits and live by them. In the past, we have been known to exercise for 10 hours straight, but we don't do that anymore. We limit ourselves to doing cardio and strength training for two hours, seven days a week. We realize that this amount still falls out of the recommended and acceptable range—and we do not advise it—but that's what we feel comfortable with at this point in our recovery. We're not bragging, either. It's pretty pathetic when exercise becomes a priority above going to church or having dream dates. But that amount of activity allows us to function for the rest of the day. And we live one day at a time...

Q   *What inspired you to become interested in health, nutrition and fitness?*

A   We were offered partial track and academic scholarships to college. Then, the obsession with food raised its ugly head, and we subsequently became curious about sports and nutrition. It was a natural tie-in. We were probably looking for the "secret diet" when we began studying these topics. We're still fascinated by new trends and stay abreast of trade journals and alternative research.

Q   *Does calorie counting work? How many calories a day do you need?*

A   The most important things to realize is if you take in more calories than you need (to work, exercise, run after your kids, etc.) from food, you will store those extra calories as fat. The reverse is also true: If you expend more energy (calories) in a day than you take in as food, you will lose body weight. Energy in versus energy out is the proper and balanced equation.

The calorie strategies commonly quoted are not always accurate: To lose one pound of fat, you have to lose/burn/work off 3,500 calories. That's fine to dissect or study in a lab, but a calorie doesn't always equal a calorie, doesn't always equal a calorie, and so on. For example, an apple consisting of 90 calories does not nutritionally (or energy-wise) equal a donut consisting of 90 calories. The body uses and eliminates whole, fresh foods more efficiently and quickly than man-made crap. A piece of fruit is less likely to be turned into fat.

As for our own calorie intake, we become fatigued and sick when we dip below 1,000 calories a day. Two thousand calories a day usually maintains your weight if you are active. But calorie consumption varies according to your body weight, food portion, quality of food, leisure activity, exercise level and hunger drive.

Q   *How do you eat when you travel?*

A   Prior to recovery, we usually starved before our jobs and binged after. Today, we call the airlines and hotels ahead of time and request menus. Many airlines, hotels and restaurants will provide special diets for diabetics or vegetarians. Most restaurants also have excellent choices of protein, vegetables and fruit. Ask your waiter how your meal is cooked, and if it can be grilled or steamed without oil or heavy sauces. When in doubt — in airport cafeterias — always bring your own fruit, hardboiled eggs, nuts and juice.

Q   *In recovery, how do you resist the influence of people who don't eat properly?*

A   Usually, we gravitate towards successful, disciplined people with fundamentally healthy appetites. It may be presumptuous, but we think we can determine a person's maturity level by their diet behavior. We have always been attracted to professional athletes, for example, and you don't see them eating too many Twinkies. We also tend to influence people around us because we are very dedicated to this way of life.

Q   *What is Kombucha Mushroom, and why's it so popular?*
A   It is both a yeast culture and bacteria and can be eaten or taken in tea form. As with other fads, the Food and Drug Administration substantiates no health claims about this mushroom. However, based on our experience, when properly fermented, the mushroom helps energy, weight loss, detoxification and alleviates intestinal problems.

Q   *What was the most fanatical diet you've tried?*
A   The most radical was fasting on distilled water and eating one orange a day for 20 days. The benefits included extreme (yet temporary) weight loss—we won't tell you how much. Absurd. Fasting felt very cleansing and rejuvenating for the first few days when we still endured the extremes. But the potential for harm was extraordinary: we lost so much muscle tissue, and our skin lost elasticity. We slowed our metabolism to a crawl since, after a few days, we didn't have the energy to exercise. Then, once we started eating again, we were insatiable and gained all of those pounds back again. It took about 40 days—double the fast period—for our energy and sleep patterns to return to normal. Not worth it!

Q   *Is hunger a result of psychological conditioning or physical predisposition?*
A   Just like in the case of alcoholism, it has been discovered that there is a gene which makes a person predisposed to be a food addict. Research has also found that normal fat cells contain leptin, a messenger hormone, which tells the hypothalamus in the brain that the body is full. In overweight people, leptin is either missing from fat cells or is dormant. Some research also indicates that one out of three overweight adults in the United States was born with biological drive to overeat.

Q   *Which foods and supplements are beneficial?*
A   The most important factor is the absence of impure food from your diet. The body is so sophisticated that it has the capacity to replace what is harmful, rid itself of unwanted toxins and rejuvenate cells.

But if the body is overworked on large amounts of non-nutritious food, it does not have the energy to detox, burn fat and heal, as well as engage in other vital functions.

Fatty Acids (and Essential Fatty Acids or EFAs) are necessary for growth and overall health. A diet high in essential fatty acids increases metabolic function and decreases body fat formation. Some fatty acids increase hormone production and increase brain functioning; some help wound healing, and some (especially primrose oil) ease PMS and menstrual symptoms. *Brewer's yeast* is comprised of the dried, pulverized cells of yeast; it is high in protein, minerals and B vitamins. It may reduce cholesterol, help wound healing and aid in the treatment of skin problems. *Vitamin B12* is beneficial for vegan vegetarians (produce only) who are missing some proteins and nutrients in their diet. *Kelp,* high in iodine, is a brown sea vegetable, which protects cells and acts as an antioxidant. *Yogurt* with acidophilus cultures helps keep the intestinal tracts clean. *Tofu* and other soy products contain natural estrogen and are beneficial before and during PMS and menopause to ease symptoms. *Wheat grass juice* is a good internal cleanser. *Wheat germ oil* (high in Vitamin E) supplies vitamins and may increase exercise performance and endurance.

Q   *What are the newest supplements we should know about?*

A   *Creatine* is a nitrogen-containing substance found in meat and fish; it's made naturally in the body. In recent research, it has been shown to increase strength and muscle mass and help prevent fatigue in active people. But read labels and take in recommended doses only. And while it's not a dietary supplement yet, there's solid new research on the amino acid compound nicknamed *SAMe* (along with folic acid and B12), used as an antidepressant. Popular in Europe for years, the combination purportedly synthesizes mood-booster brain chemicals (dopamine and serotonin) and does not cause the side effects found in common chemical antidepressants. *Valerian root* is a powerful herb good for treating insomnia, stress, gas and menstrual cramps; improper doses may cause depression.

Q   *Should I eat lighter at night?*

A   Depends on your diet and activity level. Let's put it this way: if you eat a 2,000-calorie breakfast (for example) and nothing else all day—but you stayed active—you'd probably lose weight because you utilized all those calories throughout the day. On the contrary, if you ate nothing during the rest of the day but ate a 2,000-calorie dinner at night, you might gain weight. Your metabolism would slow without calories during the day, and you wouldn't burn 2,000 calories effectively as you slept. To boost metabolism, keep blood sugar steady and maintain smart eating patterns, never skip breakfast calories, and eat most of your food during morning and afternoon meals, when you still have the chance to burn off those calories.

Q *Do men and women gain weight differently?*

A Yes. Men usually gain weight first around the abdomen, which gives them a protruding belly and a spare tire around their middle. Women have the tendency to gain weight first on their hips, legs and midriff, which is shown to be a safer place to gain weight, since abdominal fat is directly linked to heart disease. Men also have a tendency to gain weight inside, around their organs, as opposed to women, who gain weight on the outside. Therefore, a man could be fatally obese at a lower weight point, than a woman could. Eating too much processed food can also make the intestines to drop, showing a bigger stomach. This is from the lack of muscle use in the stomach and intestines, which are normally used when digesting wholesome foods with fiber.

Q *What are some common side effects of losing a significant amount of weight?*

A You might first feel lightheaded due to decreased blood pressure, and you'll be dehydrated from the loss of electrolytes. Fatigue, irritation, constipation, as well as diarrhea, are other common complaints. Anytime you change your diet, your body must gradually adjust. Be sure to drink plenty of water, eat at least 25-30 grams of fiber per day and maintain an exercise regimen.

Q *When I over-train, I taste salt in my mouth and feel salty residue on my clothes. Is this normal?*

A Taking any medication or diuretics interferes with the natural process of losing weight and may cause strange taste sensations. But what you probably taste is the body's loss of electrolytes (lots of sodium in these minerals). Some athletes who use mostly anaerobic energy (hockey and tennis players, for instance) report salty deposits in their mouth, too. A special note: The armpit is an emergency cooling organ and salty excretions or smells may also indicate stress or an unhealthy diet.

Q *Is there hope for a person who has been obese her whole life?*

A Of course. Proper diet and adequate movement can benefit anyone at any age—it's never too late to start living well. Slow, proper weight loss — in 1-2 pound weekly increments—should be accompanied by regular exercise. Food consistency is more important than the severity of the meal plan. Depending on how overweight you are to start with, you might join an organized program or get dietary supervision to get going. Do not start tomorrow—start today—and cultivate daily support from friends and loved ones. We know you can do it.

Q   *What is cellulite?*

A   There are many theories about cellulite, which we covered in the Fat Chapter. The most common prevention route is exercise; and the younger you start training, the less cellulite you'll accumulate. Other reasons for frustrating fatty deposits may be poor circulation, a sedentary lifestyle and genetic predisposition. (But very skinny supermodels often have cellulite—and that's all about genetics.) Cellulite is probably 80 percent genetic bad luck and 20 percent — lifestyle choices.

Q   *How do meditation and affirmations aid weight loss?*

A   The body is moving energy, and the power of our mind dictates the way our bodies work. Deep breathing, meditation and positive thinking all enhance our body's programming. Also, stress and tension will overwork stress hormones, tighten our muscles, weaken the immune system, cause insomnia and un-focus our attention on our body and mind. Meditation can keep the body balanced, lower blood pressure and ease the tensions of the day.

Q   *Is it true that you gain weight easier when you get older?*

A   Sort of. First, your overall lifestyle tends to become more sedentary as you age. (It, of course, does not have to end up this way.) Biologically, our metabolic rate slows slightly as we age, and it seems harder to shed pounds with each decade. However, proper diet and a consistent fitness program can neutralize the furtive effects of aging. Wholesome foods, weight training and regular aerobics can help you feel younger and sexier, too.

Q   *I'm confused. Is it better to lift heavy weights with few repetitions or light weights with high repetitions?*

A   Both. Use light weights with high repetitions (using 12-15 repetitions per set) to build muscular endurance, and use heavier weights (do 8-12 reps) to build muscular strength. Variety is the key: A well-rounded fitness program using different equipment, various exercises and diverse lifting techniques will help you sculpt the best body ever.

Q   *Do you believe in drinking at least 8-10 glasses of water a day? What's better — distilled or regular?*

A   New studies prove that the thirst mechanism kicks in noticeably when dehydration has already begun. However, if you learn to be in tune with your body, your sensitivity to thirst will increase. In such case, drink only when you are thirsty. However, do not overdo it. Drinking too much can overload the bladder and even cause edema. Or too much water can act as a diuretic washing away the minerals in the body that enable the water-hold. If you are too thirsty, this is a sign that your kidneys are washing away toxins (alcohol, stress, caffeine, medications, excess vitamins, etc.) When we binged, we were chronically thirsty. Some experts believe that you can't overload your bladder with excess water; yet, try running a marathon after drinking gallons of water, and you'll be cursing those experts every mile or so. Many fasting institutions prefer distilled water, so that minerals do not accumulate. However, many people object to distilled water because it can leach the body's own minerals (causing mineral depletion, which, in turn, will cause dehydration). Also, bottled or filtered water is better than tap water.

Q   *If someone is not a laxative abuser, do you approve of natural laxatives, enemas or colonics to enhance evacuation?*

A   A nutritious, consistent diet will eventually repair your body's natural evacuation problems. Every time you "help" out your body via enemas or laxatives, you weaken it and make it dependent on the medications. Contrary to popular belief: you do not simply flush away toxins in a colonic. Friendly bacteria in the lower intestine, which are very important for evacuation, are also flushed away. So what happens? You become constipated and have to repeat the cycle. Too much fiber (generally over 35 grams per day) can also cause constipation. Constipation or irregular bowel movement are often warning signs of a poor diet, side effects from drugs or medications, hormonal imbalances (especially during the menstrual cycle) stress or sickness. Natural laxatives may not have the dangerous chemicals that synthetic laxatives do, but laxatives in general are unhealthy. Again, constipation is not a problem; it's a symptom.

Q   *Do you eat fat-free snacks?*

A   Eating fat does not automatically make you fat. Over-indulging in anything—carbohydrates, protein, or fat—makes you fat. However, consuming lots of simple, sugary snacks is the worst even if they're fat-free as it can cause insulin overflow from the pancreas, which interferes with fat and carbohydrate metabolism. As we've stated before, excess of any nutrient which is not utilized by the body will be stored as fat.

Q   *Do you dine at restaurants now? How do you maintain a healthy nutritional regimen?*

A   We like simple health food eateries. We are no longer vegetarians, but we eat very little chicken and fish. We prefer raw fruit and vegetables, whole grains, tofu, beans and nuts. Desserts are either simple sprouted sweet breads or yogurt mixed with fruit. If we eat junk, it is like getting drunk. We no longer crave it, except to get high, so we stay away. We make our own juices and vegetable drinks daily.

We are like the Terminator—we can scan a restaurant menu and have a digital brain printout of the total calories in ten seconds. Yes, we do eat out occasionally but the waiters don't like us by the end of the order! All restaurants have simple meats and fish, vegetables and fruit. It is the sauces, dressings and side dishes that make the food despoiled of nutrients. Do not be afraid to ask the waiter about the ingredients and how the meal is cooked.

We do not count grams or calories; we go by common sense, hunger and portion size, and we choose nature's foods rather than man-made snacks. Counting calories, fat grams, and weighing yourself keeps you body-obsessed. You know intuitively what you should eat or not; so ask yourself if you want it badly enough.

Q   *Where is the best place to learn about diets and nutrition?*

A   We classify nutrition with politics and religion—a very controversial and emotional topic. Every month, new fads and news articles completely contradict those of the month before. Ask a well-read registered dietician at a university or hospital for advice on the newest food fad or supplement. We've experimented with everything, and we're open to new trends, but we think that body intuition is the best teacher.

Q   *How can you tell if you're taking too many vitamins, or if your diet is right for you?*

A   Urine should be clear. When our urine is green-ish, it's from excess vitamins or unabsorbed nutrients. If urine is yellow, it is from excess waste, dieting bingeing or even too much exercise. If your urine is brown, there's something seriously wrong. See your doctor. The bowel movements should be light, but not too light; very light bowel coloring is a sign of liver problem. Fecal matter should come out with ease — at least once a day — hardly needing any cleaning. Dark bowels are a sign of excess protein or carbs in the diet and sometimes represent old fecal matter. Constipation is a result of eating heavy meals of refined carbs or too much protein. Women have a third way of cleaning up - our periods. The heavier the diet - the thicker the lining in the uterus. A light period means a clean diet.

Always remember that too much of a particular vitamin or food can deplete the body of some other nutrient it desperately needs. Variety and moderation keep the body in a perfect condition.

Q *Why do women seem to gain weight faster than men?*

A First, men have more muscles, and muscle tissue is more active. Women store fat more efficiently for childbearing and beyond. We are also born with more fat cells. Finally, our history may be responsible, if we look at it in simple terms: during the prehistoric age, men ventured out and hunted for survival while women cared for the young a home and literally kept those home fires burning. Men purportedly craved more protein because they needed it for muscle repair. Women craved foods which kept them padded with fat, since fat was needed to keep them warm (fat cells are insulation akin to a windbreaker). Even studies today prove that women tend to naturally eat more fat and carbohydrates while men consume more protein.

The Hollywood lifestyle

Q *How do you compare your real persona with your image?*

A Our image was invented and packaged for fans to interpret. We are commonly referred to as sexy parodies or social enigmas (not very flattering). These days we do not describe ourselves, we just ARE ourselves. Maybe for the very first time ever.

Q *Do other models and actresses have food disorders and hide it?*

A It's not a good recovery practice to pick through other people's emotional inventory when we still have so much work to do ourselves. But you can imagine that the pressure and body obsession caused by the media would turn any "normy" into someone who needs dysfunctional escape. (Some social experts would say that just about one in every three people in this town suffers from disordered eating and body dysmorphic disorder.)

Drugs, alcohol and food disorders are prevalent in all domains, not just in modeling and acting. But because the media focuses on Hollywood bodies so much, maybe we notice them more here. Anonymity is an important factor in sobriety, so we'll respect that and move to the next question.

Q *Did show biz and modeling hasten your disease?*

A We have modeled on and off since we were seven years

old. Yet, even before that we remember worrying that we were too heavy to ride our horses! We learned to suppress our feelings with food and to control our lives with bulimia from a very early age. So, perhaps, the industry sped us along on our sickly path, but the disease was already in place.

Q   *Who do you blame for your disease?*

A   My sister ... just a co-dependent joke! Really, recovery is about stopping the blame and turning away from being a victim. It is about empowering yourself by surrendering your power. As long as we are blaming, we are not working out a solution. At this point, we do not blame anyone or anything for our disease; we are grateful to have had the chance to shape up the rest of our lives. When we are mindful of being grateful, it is a daily inventory spot-check.

Q   *Are you sorry for going the cliché route of centerfold pin-ups?*

A   We think that all adventures, experiences and mistakes make one a complete person. We are grateful to our corporate sponsors and fans for making us top sellers! Why should we bite the hand that fed us? Yet, on the other hand, we wish women would have more of a choice and a voice. We can only do this by empowering good role models, not by attacking other women.

Q   *Who are your Hollywood role models?*

A   Oprah Winfrey and Joan Rivers. They not only divulged their eating disorders, but they also confessed other heartbreaking "life issues." (Rivers had to cope with her husband's suicide; whereas Oprah told the world about her childhood sexual abuse. Heavy!) Both have also spoken candidly about their food and diet problems. Princess Diana was also a classy, dignified role model who had anorexia... She used the podium of her fame to do charity work and affect millions of people. Her contributions changed the world.

Q   *What would you advise an aspiring model or actress with a food disorder?*

A   Most young girls, not just models, obsess over body addictions, scary diets and fast fixes in order to look good. We do not encourage a practicing food addict or anorexic to expose herself to casting calls. We strongly suggest recovery first. Besides, emphasis should be on education, creative abilities, and the use of young bodies as vehicles for sports or social contribution.

Q   *Is there anything about Hollywood that still appeals to you?*

A   Hollywood is a powerful podium, the greatest place to get an important message out. What makes a difference to us is "coming out" with our bulimia. We will not forget the first time we learned the true power of the media. We had just finished a radio show, and a man came up to us, not to ask for our autograph, but to thank us for saving his sister's life. We had given her hope by sharing our insane diet stories. She quickly admitted herself to a hospital and joined a twelve-step program. She no longer considered suicide. We felt so fortunate to be involved.

Disease and recovery

Q   *What is a healthy day for you?*

A   We try to sleep for eight hours and eat three meals and two healthy snacks every day. We try to keep exercise down to a semi-normal two hours a day, surrendering a day here or there for rest. We like to read, especially books on self-help and philosophy. Our mornings start off with meditation, a vitamin/mineral juice cocktail and a jog. That keeps our bodies, minds and souls running smoothly. Daily, we aim to do recovery therapy, twelve-step meetings, workshops and charity work and to attend church.

Q   *How do you know if you are an addict?*

A   An addiction manifests when brain chemicals change, when dopamine becomes depleted and when behavior becomes distorted. You become compulsive about practicing your disease at any cost, and it's hard to practice "delayed gratification" (like waiting for dessert after dinner). There are no boundaries or regulations that say "stop" or "enough," and you do not necessarily ingest your "drug" to relax or enjoy it anymore; you do it to avoid crashing or having a crisis. Here is a situation that would qualify you as an addict: you abuse your "drug of choice" and cause a tragedy or damage to yourself or others. Normal people relate their "addiction" to this tragedy and quit. But addicts cannot quit, even when they desperately want to.

Q   *Are addicts weak people?*

A   On the contrary, they are often the most sensitive, creative people. But, once they're in the full-blown disease, they lose these qualities, as well as their own identity. We are attracted to recovering addicts because these brilliant people develop empathy, profound wisdom and humility while working towards their sobriety.

Q   *How do you help a loved one with a severe eating disorder?*

A   That depends on your relationship with them, the level of their disease and their willingness to receive help. They have to be willing, or it won't happen.

Most of all, get educated. There are recovery meetings for both addicts and co-addicts (people directly in contact with and influenced by addicts.) Self-help sections in bookstores have a lot of new and in-depth research information, and there's group therapy for people who are related to or involved with the addict.

You must never try to "control" or "fix" the sick person. You can make them aware of your concern or their negative effect on others because of their addiction. But if you don't do it carefully, you can actually make the addict revert back to isolation and into deeper depression. Denial, or pretending the problem does not exist, is not an answer, either. Intervention with both friends and family, and a qualified specialist, is the best way to address the problem and start treatment.

Q   *What is the most misconstrued aspect of recovery?*

A   THERE IS NO CURE. More importantly, recovery is a process, not an event. And there is no logic to the disease. That is why non-addicts have a hard time attempting to help addicts. Non-addicts use logic to counsel people who suffer with addiction, and there are NO logical explanations to these obsessions.

Q   *Is it better to rough it alone, or be influenced by friends and family when struggling with recovery?*

A   <u>Discriminate, do not isolate</u>! You should be surrounded by healthy people, calm places, true friends and concerned family members. Sometimes it may be best to avoid "slippery" or "trigger" areas like family dinners. Solitude is good for introspection, but old bullshit can overwhelm new wisdom.

Q   *What is the difference between therapy and twelve-step programs?*

A   Therapy is talking to someone who is qualified to listen, but might not be able to identify. Twelve-step programs are excellent for recovering addicts who work on positive solutions, and on how to deal with pain and problems of obsession.

Q   *You talk about addictions as "progressive diseases" and you also mention "functional addicts." What's the difference?*

A   The actual disease is not the act of indulging. An overeater (or a lush) can't always be classified as an addict in the disease. Compulsion is "thirst" that can never be quenched, and that's what makes the disease progressive.

Someone can be a "functional substance abuser" or an overweight overeater, and not necessarily be compulsive enough to cause severe destruction or death. They can carry on a semblance of a normal lifestyle: work hard, bond with their kids, play tennis with friends and be classified as "functional."

Q   *Why are eating disorders more prevalent with women?*

A   One obvious reason is the media. Women have to put up with the society plastering perfect (or perfectly altered) women all over the place, and be complacent with the few male sex symbols who may be sexy, as well as balding, pot-bellied aging men who are viewed as desirable. There is obviously a societal gender imbalance, and women get the short end of that stick every time. Plus, women are very emotional and very competitive. In an ideal world, women would try to stop competing or buying into the physical frenzy of perfection. They should give their vote and money to more positive role models.

Q   *How are cravings related to addiction?*

A   Good question. It often comes down to chemistry, to the unhealthy secretion of chemical messengers like dopamine, serotonin and norepinephrine, and the body's ability to regulate them. To treat it simply—and it's not a simple process—dopamine and norepinephrine are chemicals that make you feel alert and energized, and serotonin is a chemical that makes you feel smooth and mellow when your body and mind function normally. People with eating disorders have bodies and brains that do not function normally.

Q   *What was the most painful experience that prompted your recovery?*

A   Shane barfed on her lobster bib at a trendy restaurant with a famous date ... and she did not care. Quite honestly, there was not one single event that shamed us into action. It was scary not caring about anything at all; we were utterly reckless.

A real low point was when I overdosed on laxatives and was lying on the ground trying to puke out the poison, and everything hurt so much. Basically, we bottomed out by just getting sick and tired of being sick and tired.

Personal and miscellaneous questions

Q   *How do you explain your food disorder to dates or new friends?*

A   We do not. We only share it with other twelve-steppers, if they ask. (But everyone will know now!)

Q   *What work are you most proud of?*

A   Nothing. What a dilemma. We had no desire to be famous models, and our career took off when some horrible, unprofessional test shots were sent to a calendar company. Shame over our sudden fame and money made us hide, eat and purge. Now we use our experiences as opportunities for growth (no pun intended) and find that our recovery is our greatest success and that of which we're most proud. We hope to share this work with others who still suffer.

Q   *What recovery resources are available? Did you use them?*

A   There are amazing institutions, like OA, which specialize in food disorders. There are also workshops and inspirational tapes produced by John Bradshaw and Tony Robbins. We know that the problem is not just about the food, but about hidden, suppressed pain and other issues. So, we devour books on philosophy and self-help, such as those by Deepak Chopra, Parmahansa Yogananda, Mary Ann Williamson, Dr. Christian Northrup, etc. We are avid non-fiction readers, and love to browse through bookstore shelves.

Q   *Who's been instrumental in your career and recovery?*

A   We wish we could say God and Mother Teresa, but all we can say is "karma." Our career took off with us scratching our heads. Our recovery stems from a combination of loving family example, God's bountiful gifts and grudging self-acceptance.

Q   *Do you think you're role models?*

A   We hope not. But, unfortunately, almost every visible celebrity becomes an involuntary role model. That's why I think it is our responsibility to educate young people about choices, so that one specific image won't be the dictating role model of the month. We do not have to strive to be like what we see and enjoy, as those quasi-pleasing images and ideals are merely some of manifold choices available to us.

If there were one thing we'd like to be remembered for (as role models); it would be the fact that we blazed our own trail contrary to other people's negativity and skepticism. Young people should learn to work on their own unique attributes, rather than on cloning themselves to be like other starlets.

Q   *Do men care about your weight or food disorder?*

A   Most men do not understand it, and they don't notice details like women do. They see the overall blonde package, you know… A man who is into you will be open-minded, and he will be respectful and honestly attracted to the real you. Something we have learned, though, is that if you're uncomfortable with your body, then he will also learn to be uncomfortable. For every man who does not like your "type" or body weight, there is a man who does. But the real question is: Do YOU like your type?

Q   *What kind of men do you find attractive?*

A   We just love men, and they happen to come in all forms. We are attracted to real masculine strength, which is often manifested in courage and confidence, rather than muscle. But we flaunt a weakness for athletes and cowboys. The type of guy we'd "hoot" and holler at is someone who oozes masculinity. But our tastes do change to fit the man we love. You see profound wisdom in the eyes of someone who has been to Hell and back, too; so we're also attracted to men in all kinds of recovery.

Q   *Is there a difference in addiction between twins; did you binge, purge and recover together?*

A   Yes, we were Siamese Twins practicing our disease. In a recent study on twins, researchers found that the youngest twin indulges more in her disease 80 percent of the time. (It figures. I'm younger by three minutes!) But the younger twin is usually more hell-bent on recovery (right on!) I did seem to dive into the disease and recovery more than Shane does, but she disagrees. Part of the disease is to think no one is as bad as you, including your clone!

Q   *What is more dominant, nature or nurture, when it comes to healthy living?*

A   New research with twins (ironically) claims that both separated twins and twins living together are dominated 80 percent by genes and 20 percent by lifestyle. I disagree. Everything depends on the lifestyle. The more radical or extreme the lifestyle, the more it will constitute the impact on you as compared to your genes. There's a saying, which holds true, "take care of what Mother Nature gives you before Father Time takes it away." Father Time is "age," and your aging process is mostly determined by your lifestyle. Some people may have to be more conservative with respect to their lifestyle because their genes do not permit excesses easily tolerated by others. Nonetheless, I have realized better results from strict nutritional programs rather than from relying on genetic gifts.

Q   *Do you believe that anti-depressants, such as Prozac, Pazil and Zoloff, are effective for eating disorders?*

A   These drugs are useful for some; they work by stimulating your own brain neuro-transmitters to produce serotonin (the hormone in the brain which is responsible for feeling satiated, complacent, calm, etc.) and other mood-leveling drugs. Some people do need the medical jumpstart to begin living a happy, healthy life. Some may call it "cheating," or not using your own willpower or endurance. But, if your addiction is killing you, and Prozac creates an abstinence habit, then it provides a real lifeline. I never gave Prozac a chance, but I have seen great results in many people.

Q   *Are most of your friends recovered addicts?*

A   Yes. Our companions include recovering alcoholics, compulsive overeaters, anorexics, etc. Not only do we identify with them, but we have observed them work their way up from their "bottom" to become the most non-judgmental, courageous, humble and honest people we have known. (It takes those tough qualities to attain and sustain sobriety.)

Q   *What physical effects did your eating disorder have on you?*

A   The saddest part is that we lost years of our lives in a food fog. We have also have experienced some heart damage, stomach and liver problems, chronic overuse exercise injuries (our knees and ankles are shot), and we had to bleach our teeth to restore their normal appearance.

Q   *What does it mean when people say that alcoholism, anorexia and bulimia are spiritual diseases?*

A   ˙ Those diseases are three-fold: mental, spiritual and physical. Physically, your body is dependent on your drug of choice. That is why you must "dry out" to initiate recovery. Mentally, your thinking becomes distorted, and then it's your "stinking thinking" that makes you sicker and more out of touch with reality. And then, you get to the point where willpower stops working, and only a miracle, intervention or God can help. (That's where the spiritual angle enters into the equation.) Even if you do not believe in God, you still need to surrender, strive for virtue, help others and live honest lives. Personal empowerment comes from transforming you and empowering others, and THAT happens to be very spiritual, indeed.

Chapter 14

Relationships, lies and videotape

This is the shortest chapter. Sad to say, but our energy was elsewhere for most all of our adult lives. Since our infamous images had sensual overtones, we were frequently asked on dates. What was more perplexing, was that stars had such tremendous romantic interest in us. Here we were, hot-to-trot pin-ups attracting credible celebrities—yet we felt that we had absolutely NOTHING to offer them. Dating and relationships were just like all of our photo shoots: deprivation—before and food reward—after. Nothing and no one ever felt real; our romances were as fake as the pictures for which we gladly posed.

Because of our dysfunctional childhood and our co-dependence, we tended to attract alcoholics. Shane and Sia to the rescue! Because of our mother's therapy, our past experience and schooling, we had the blessing of being able to bring our significant others into recovery; we identified with alcoholics. We did not know what a normal, loving relationship was like.

Hollywood is known for both its "isms" and for recovery. We felt a sense of irony by receiving a certain celebrity status. We learned that relationships are not in your best interest during the first years of sobriety. We were mothers, nurses or therapists. We did not know how to have balanced relationships.

We couldn't stand people who would kiss and tell, and we always respected the privacy of the celebrities we dated. We noticed that the bigger the star was, the better he treated us. We were not competition to him. And we yearned to feel love-butterflies in our stomach instead of the roar of laxatives. But love or lust kills appetite, and shame soon drove us deeper into addiction.

Most people pictured us as leading glamorous lives and having wild parties with the rich and famous. HAHAHAHAHAHAHA. Not only were most of our nights spent alone and in confusion; they were filled with deprivation, isolation and the fear of being found out. However, when you feel unworthy of a mercy date offered by a star, it's twice as embarrassing to go out with him and have the tabloids "out you" before the first mercy kiss.

We used to classify men into four categories: Down-to-earth males who wanted nothing to do with Hollywood (they were our first choice, and Shane lucked out with Ken Wahl, God bless him). Then, there were men who would grasp at date straws because they identified us as tabloid princesses. Yuck. The third category was the Hollywood celebs who used their position or fame to seek us out. Last, but certainly not least, were powerful businessmen who did not wear success on their sleeves. But their significant others were women WE would marry! That is, we felt that those strong, confident women were their perfect matches. We had no right to date a healthy, sexy normal man. We belonged to the Bermuda Triangle dating club, and that was where we stayed.

We were always attracted to athletes, though. We dated a few men who were utterly obsessed with their physicality or who were fanatical about their health and fitness. Those dates were typically limited to gyms with gigantic mirrors or to the organic isles in a health food store. Boring and psychologically unhealthy date mates for the Barbi Twins, wouldn't you say? Now we prefer men with a sense of maturity who incorporate balance, discrimination and compassion for addiction, especially if they're familiar with it.

Instead of looking for Mr. Right, I try to be grateful for the men I've dated and for the opportunity to meet others. I take it one day at a time. Just like with dieting and recovery, I surrender my dating habits to a Higher Force. I do the footwork by building my own sense of self-worth, and I know that Mr. Right will stand in front of me, someday.

Whether you are a celebrity or the girl next-door, our advice is the same: do not try to control the situation, stop fixing your dates and invest in bettering yourself. Be grateful for the peaceful process of progress; do not seek perfection. You have nothing to offer others unless you earn it first for yourself.

Again, we do not regret anything or anyone. Each new romantic experience has delivered to us another lesson to learn. When you blame someone else for a sour romance, you become a victim and cannot accept your deserved lessons. So, learn and move on, sisters.

I know that I am an addict who can transmit addiction during an intimate moment, so I keep my sensual appetite in balance with my self-investment. My attraction lies in the rapport with my loved one, and not with what he does or what he can do for me. I think you can make love way before you become intimate. And the ultimate pleasure is found in mutual joy.

Men often have this natural urge to "rescue," and some women love to be "rescued." Unfortunately, this phenomenon generates a co-dependent relationship where the man (an "enabler") rescues the woman (the "victim"), who naturally then shuns off blame and responsibility towards the rescuer. Most people with addiction are attracted to this unhealthy cycle in a relationship. A child in a healthy family learns to make choices from security and love. A child in a dysfunctional family learns to make choices from fear, hiding shame and guilt within. Having no boundaries or true childhood, she later becomes an "adult child," control freak or addict.

This pattern is, most definitely, carried out in a relationship. Some people try to repair—with their mates—what they had unresolved with their parents. A person, who was sexually abused as a child, has no sexual boundaries. Because, as a child, she felt robbed, she wants to give power to herself by taking something back. Therefore, her sex becomes her power in manipulation. She learns to hide her shame and guilt by medicating her feelings with alcohol, food or chemicals. Her relationships are always about "taking," rather than giving.

I am confident that a relationship should be equal, "give-and-take," in order to work. A healthy relationship is never about control or fixing, but is rather about allowing the other to have his or her individuality, space and respect. It takes a lot more than love to be together. It takes a lot of learning to become a better person through the tolerance of love. Relationships should help a person expand rather that isolate.

Crushes or obsessions are often confused with love, and yet they are more like addiction, rather than love. They isolate, limit and destroy. To avoid this problem, learn to let go, and let God do his will in your life. Letting go does not equal giving up; it just means trusting the Higher Power. Only when you accomplish it, you will see that your "drug of choice" (food, alcohol or chemicals) will no longer be needed. Each relationship my sister and I had taught us to commit, keep respect and do our best, a day at a time. The fastest way to destroy a relationship is to have expectations. Have none. But remember: you cannot give what you do not have yourself. So, first love yourself. Then—expand; do not close off.

Scary diet story 23

The very best love affair you can have during an eating disorder is with the telephone. When you're weak and miserable from dieting, let your fingers do the walking—right to the telephone. Or when you're bingeing, bloated and too stuffed to move, the phone is a great tool for canceling dates or continuing romance. Your lover will never see the food stains on your shirt or your milk mustache ... not if you practice your sultry 900-number voice. Having your lover on the other end of the phone while gorging your brains out is like having two simultaneous orgasms.

Then there are times when we are simply too unhappy to dress up and party. Besides, who wants to initiate a binge AND adhere to strict table manners at a fancy restaurant? The phone is a far better date—just dial; boy, we put Ma Bell's kids through college.

After one successful pre-date purge, I was left with a remarkably flat stomach, but I had red watery eyes, and breath that could annihilate an army. But I was determined not to let it ruin my night! I'd wash up, gargle and eat a small meal before we headed to dinner so that I wouldn't lose control at the table. I'd make a small salad with whatever was hanging around in the refrigerator: avocados, olive oil, carrots, tomatoes, maybe artichoke hearts. Well, a balanced meal should include protein. Eureka—a pound of cheese! Boy, was my salad beautiful, colorful, huge and ... FATTENING!

I may as well have eaten a cake with all of the calories and fat grams in that baby. It was the size of my kitchen table, for goodness sake. After I scarfed every bite, I was so bloated that I had to cancel my date, 30 minutes before he picked me up. So, back to the phone I went. When I called my date, he blurted, "Okay, who died this time?" I guess my excuses were becoming ridiculous by then.

Scary diet story 24

There's an annoying question "normies" always ask compulsive overeaters: what is it that makes you eat beyond hunger? Do you blame a flunked driver's test or do you blame not being able to understand your VCR? It's hard to translate that overwhelming passion for eating into simple words... Sometimes it's the pristine sight of pastry, the smell of baking bread or the way milk and cookies melt in your mouth.

I once had the insane idea to torch my taste buds. So I fetched the perfect "tool" for that job—burning hot food! I "nuked" my potato a little longer than usual, and, voila! A potato too hot to handle — perfect! Hmmm ... yum ... oh, oh ... my taste buds were still dancing. So back in the microwave it went! Finally, I retrieved my dilapidated, anorexic French fry and courageously ate the charcoal potato like a terrorist downing a cyanide capsule. Success! A tongue Freddy Kruger would have envied. My problem? I needed to cool down the painful flames in my mouth. What is cool and light? Cool Whip! After eight tubs of Cool Whip I knew my problem wasn't taste; it was texture. I would be sure to try chocolate next time around...

Chapter 15

The Barbis' freedom diet and health formula

1. This is not a diet! Consider it a release from the bondage of food deprivation and body obsession. Plan your meals carefully so eating well becomes a daily achievement. Do the footwork and surrender the results.

2. Your sensible regimen should consist of three meals and two snacks daily. Adhere to our nutrient ratio of about equal amounts of protein and carb calories, and half of that amount in fat. You will consume 40 percent of your daily intake in protein, 40 percent—in carbohydrates, and 20 percent—in fat calories.

3. Eat your heaviest carb meal in the AM—see our Recipe Chapter for ideas. Don't deprive—replace! For every refined sugar pastry, there is a natural sweet alternative, for every saturated or bad fat there is a helpful fat (for example: replace butter with olive oil, or nut butter).

4. Take special care not to eat when you are upset; or two hours before bedtime; when you are just not hungry; when you are very sick; or as part of a false reward system.

5. Don't deprive—replace! Substitute every refined sugar snack with a healthier, sweet alternative. (Swap fruit for cookies, and cereal bars—for candy and cake.) Replace saturated or "bad" fats with "good" fats (for example, swap butter for olive oil).

6. Eat at least 25 grams per day of what we call "broom foods," raw and fibrous vegetables, legumes, peas, lentils and grains.

7. You are entitled to one "no-no treat" each day, but make sure that the snack has some redeeming qualities. For instance: If you have ice

cream, sprinkle vitamin-rich nuts on top; or if you have a slice of cheesy pizza, add mushrooms, peppers or other veggies. Also, it's best to eat your "no-no treat" one hour after exercise when appetite is reduced and metabolism is revving right along.

8. Put food deposits in the bank for emergency withdrawals if you plan to travel or be away from home for long. Bring your food journal, a great pair of exercise shoes and prepare a mental list of the foods that will quench your desire to binge. When the familiar feeling hits, you'll be prepared. I call this "allowed-disallowed" eating. I know my "trigger" foods that set me in a binge. But planning and writing it down, rather than waiting for the treat makes me saner and less compulsive.

9. Regular cardio, strength and flexibility exercise will curb appetite, burn fat, boost your energy and clear the body of toxins and the mind of negativity. Pick a pal who will walk, jog or in-line skate with you, at least three times per week.

10. Don't weigh yourself or count specific calories or fat grams. Eat smaller portions of wholesome, balanced foods. Listen to your body's intuition; you inherently know what your body needs, more than any expert does. Enjoy the process and the brand-new way of looking at food and fitness.

The more natural a food is, the less the protein/carb/fat ratio is important. For example, nuts are a perfect snack—with protein, carbs and fat present—but they have more fat and carbs than protein. The 40-40-20 ratio varies according to time of day, amount of workout, types of food and, especially, the fat content.

In the morning my carb intake is higher; after a good workout I have my treats, and at night I have heavier protein- and fat-containing meals, such as an avocado/tuna salad. The Barbis' freedom diet combines a number of great diets, but it also uses your intuition and incorporates more variation. For example, Dr. Barry Sears, author of The Zone Diet advises the ratio of 30-40-40. The Barbis' freedom diet changes the ratio to 40-40-20, with the allowance for variation, according to a particular person's needs.

When you lose your appetite or crave carbs, you may be eating too much protein. If you're bloated, fatigued or dissatisfied, you may be consuming too many carbs, especially when it's weighed against your fat intake. And if you have glandular or hormonal problems (like wild mood swings or extreme irritability) your fat intake may be too high OR too low.

More questions and answers

Editor's note: These questions and answers were reprinted (practically unedited) from the actual Barbi Twins' online sessions on E! Television and Entertainment Tonight websites.

Q   *How many calories should a person consume a day?*

A   Research shows that in order to maintain weight you should be eating 10 calories per pound of body weight. However, we believe that it is really dependent upon your personalized factors.

Q   *How long have you been in recovery? Do you think you're cured?*

A   Thank God there is no "cure" or it would turn into another unpleasant "fix." Recovery is an ongoing progress enabling different facets of our lives—in order to keep the reward... sobriety! The bonuses are peace and fulfillment combined with humility and gratefulness.

Q   *How would you compare yourselves to your image?*

A   We feel that we've been enmeshed, dysfunctional, co-dependent addicts who can't look in the mirror. Quite honestly, our image was "packaged" for the fans to interpret on their own. We are referred to as sexy parodies or enigmas. But we would just describe ourselves as "us ... just being us!"

Q   *If there's one thing you could change, what would it be?*

A   What a question to ask a controlling, perfection-driven co-dependent! We've got a Christmas list. But in our recovery we're learning that nothing is a mistake. The best quote I've heard was "God, please do not change my circumstances, help me change my outlook on them." Every obstacle is like a barbell at a gym to strengthen the "muscle" of discrimination and empathy. So, while my disease wants to change everything, my recovery uses my experiences to change my attitude and to attain the feeling of gratitude. (Although I guess I could not have minded being the firstborn—instead of my bossy sis!)

Q *As part of your recovery, what was the most difficult thing to give up?*

A I think sugar was the hardest to give up. I enjoyed it so much. Yet, it was the "trigger" food that caused an out-of-control anxiety. Giving up the most loved treat turned into the biggest relief. We had to accept that our eating habits were not normal—we had a disease. At first we fought the notion of being bulimic, trying to exercise our willpower and to prove to ourselves that we merely need "moderation." But surrendering made it easier for us. We just accepted the disease and put our energy into full recovery, rather than into white-knuckling the abstinence.

Q *What was the most painful experience that you endured in your recovery up to now?*

A When I found out my sister had recovery six minutes before me. No, I think it was trying to quit the business when the business would not let us quit. It made us look like irresponsible drug addicts when we did not turn up for jobs—even though they had been booked without our permission or originally declined. Our co-dependence and people-pleasing would push us into doing a half-ass job, ruining our image, when in actuality we just wanted to take a break and come back when we took control of our disease and were ready. Finally, we just stopped working. We took a four-year break to go through recovery and to obtain degrees in nutrition. So, at this point, we do not "sell our mistakes" anymore; we "blaze our own trail," at our own pace. One project at a time, one day at a time.

Q *Your books and interviews advise people what to do. What advice would you give to someone to NEVER do?*

A Diet! It is a perceived solution, which invariably turns into a real problem. Every overweight person I've known has dieted and has become even heavier. Dieting attacks the symptom, not the core issue—the cause of the food disorder. And for a severely overweight person with a real medical problem dieting is the worst enemy. It would make her condition even worse.

Proper nutrition (not crazy dieting) will work for most people if they complete steps in recovery—mentally, spiritually and physically. A food disorder is a threefold disease, not just a physical affliction. The obsession with wanting to be thin will turn into an obsession with crazy dieting. Nip it in the bud and work on the root; do not just prune the leaves.

Q   *Is there more recovery or disease in your family?*

A   Let's put it this way, we're not the Waltons, we're the Addams Family; but we are proud of it. We have big-time, real recovery in our family; we have family members practicing "isms," as well. We even have some "normies." But everyone respects each other's path. The "ism" of the disease is proven to be genetic. We had heredity working against us. We also saw vivid examples of "drowning" the pain. But the examples of sobriety glowed through the darkest of the nights. And were most powerful, thank God.

Q   *What was the most flattering event or picture of you?*

A   As we said before, we were in our full-fledged disease during our work period, and it showed in our faces and health. The disease also made us feel shame. That shame drew sharks who produced lousy products to sell to our fans. Yet, our "image" became a household name around the world.

Q   *Do you like your image to represent sexiness or health and athleticism?*

A   I think athletic and healthy is sexy. If we had it our way, we would not have had our photos posed in beds. It is cliché. We would rather have our pictures taken while we are exercising on step machines. A pumped bicep and quadricep is more interesting than the predictable cleavage shot.

Q   *You say that you are turned off by Hollywood. What do you mean?*

A   As we said before, our products were mass-produced with poor quality. Since we did modeling, our print images were our bread and butter, our work. No matter how good we could have looked in person, one missing element ruined our look in print. We didn't hear, "I'm sorry the color scanner did not work well," or "the printer made a mistake." Instead, we would hear, "I'm sorry you looked bad." And our fans were ripped off. What I also noticed was that women are revered more for looks than men. And unlike men, it seems that women are more competitive with each other. They do not enjoy the camaraderie men have. Some women either attack other women or try to "one-up" them, usually via looks and physicality. When notions like "inner beauty is more important" or "develop a talent" are preached but not practiced, young girls get a hypocritical message. If you were to survey most young girls asking what they aspire to be, who they admire or even remember, they will recall models and popular bathing suit pinups, not athletes, scientists or good actresses who trained hard for their profession. This situation is a turnoff for Shane and me, which is especially poignant with respect to our reentry to the entertainment world.

Q   *Which nutritional motto would you endorse?*

A   Food is not a cure! It is a way of life! You are as healthy as you eat. That's the same with diets. It should be a routine way of life. Once you "finish" a diet and go back to "normal" or familiar eating habits, your weight and health problems will return, as well. Cultivate good eating habits, and your weight and health will always be what they should be.

Q   *Which is worse: to be a drug addict/alcoholic or a bulimic/compulsive overeater?*

A   There's no one way of answering that. If you are using hardcore drugs and alcohol, you will kill yourself or destroy your health very fast. Moreover, a drug addict usually has poor eating habits. Anorexia, bulimia and compulsive overeating can kill just as easily, depending on how bad the destructive behavior is. Abusing laxatives is a drug abuse. They contain ephedrine, as well as other dangerous chemicals. Although there are studies that starving rats live longer, that test was to prove that small amounts of fuel are better utilized than an overabundance. Complete abstinence from food, especially when active, is "enervating" (nerve energy utilized) and will eventually tear down your vital tissue, weaken your immune system, and can kill you. But from my observation, I have noticed that diet and food abusers, especially overweight victims, wear more destruction on the face and body than people in alcohol recovery. Going up and down in weight and carrying too much extra weight is extremely tiring on the body. You really can't compare the two diseases with such a relative question.

Q   *How do you know which are the best ingredients when dietary research is so controversial? Example: margarine and butter. Which is your first choice: diet foods (with fructose, artificial sweeteners, etc.) or health food that may be fattening?*

A   I always say that you can't go wrong with organic food in its natural state—the way we are meant to eat it. I'm reluctant when it comes to new or artificial, "fake," shortcuts such as fat or sugar substitutes. After years of thinking margarine is better than butter, came the discovery of trans-fatty acids (the by-product from hydrogenating oil to a solid form). These trans-fatty acids do more harm than does the fat in butter. Sugar is like a drug to my sister and me; it destroys the insulin balance, increases one's set point in weight, has an addictive nature, is a proven depressant, etc. Marijuana and hashish are "natural" and, yet, not healthy. Meats are unnaturally raised—with a lot of hormones and chemicals. And artificial sweeteners are constantly discovered to have new side effects (for example, excitotoxins, a by-product of artificial sweeteners or an overload of carbs, cause brain damage and promote serious disorders, such as Alzheimer's and Parkinson's diseases). Fructose is said to be the only sugar that does not cause an insulin overflow. However, it is true for those with insulinemia and those who are prone to edema or are sugar sensitive. Pulp in fruit helps the insulin balance and fructose assimilation. The body either recognizes something as a food or as a drug/poison. The farther the food is from its natural state (overcooked, over-cut or oxidized or in any way changed), the less the body will utilize it. Fruit and vegetables are best raw or slightly steamed, and should dominate your diet along with clean, simple protein foods. Diet foods are absurd. They stress low calories and incorporate artificial ingredients. Healthy foods are <u>not</u> fattening in simple natural forms: small portions of nuts, avocados, seeds, etc.

Q   *Do overweight people have low metabolism?*

A   We go into great detail in the book about how to fix slow metabolism to help reduce body fat. Surprisingly, however, studies show that people are often overweight due to excess eating, which raises their metabolism! Most overweight people do not have low metabolism. Recent research has shown that only 5% of overweight people have naturally low metabolism. Same research also found that the real culprit of the excess weight is dormant leptin—the hormone responsible for fat control on a cellular level. If an overweight person has low metabolism, it is from starving combined with bingeing, which made their bodies fat-efficient. Any time an overweight person with normally high metabolism acquires slow metabolism, it is due to dieting—in any form.

Q   *Which do you recommend: vegetable or animal protein?*

A   Vegetable protein is packaged together with vegetable fiber which combination slows the protein absorption into the bloodstream. Animal protein does not come with fiber, which makes it more absorbable. It is interesting that many religions prohibit meat eating in order to stay clean for praying, as historically meat contained many parasites. Modern-day meat is, by and large, safe from parasites, but it contains a load of hormones and antibiotics (and let's forget pesticides and herbicides which are neatly packaged into the food cows eat—passed on to us in meat). Eating pork is considered dangerous by some worshippers, because pigs can eat poison without dying, but pass it on to us. Moreover, vegetable protein is better digested and does not come packaged with saturated fat. For those and other reasons, I prefer a variety of vegetable protein sources. I incorporate some meat into my diet, as long as it is lean and is organically raised, without antibiotics and hormones.

Q   *Therapists and self-help books tell you to love yourself, love your inner child, and to make those affirmations, looking in a mirror. Do you agree or practice this?*

A   I'd usually smash the mirror. Joking aside, as corny as it seems, it is important to love yourself (or your inner child, as some refer to it). That may be very difficult to do when you're close to suicide or are in a very destructive stage. It may feel phony or mechanical. I think you have to build up self-worth in order to feel good about yourself. The mirror is hard to look at if your body-obsession is the focus of your disease. Self-worth comes in being productive, disciplined in commitments, and making contributions. Then at some stage you can pick up the mirror and see your inner beauty manifest through your eyes.

Q   *Why are some people's addictions worse than those of others?*

A   A lot of reasons. Are you genetically prone? Did your role models have dysfunctional behavior? Do you live in denial? And besides, for many people, the same amount of dopamine (pleasure brain chemical) is excreted in anticipation of an experience as that during the actual experience. This phenomenon creates "cravings." This can make someone be compulsive, and not practice delayed gratification (waiting for the appropriate time). They indulge in the experience they remembered. This creates addiction. The more dopamine, the stronger the addiction probability.

Q   *Can poor health be reversed?*

A   Yes. Not only can you supply depleted nutrients, you can both repair past damage and prevent future damage. Although I think that proper nutrition is more powerful than drugs, it is not a magical cure. It is a way of life. It is like being in remission. As long as you clean up your diet (the cleaner the diet, the healthier you become) and consistently maintain your good diet and fitness lifestyle (along with fresh air, sunshine and stress relievers like meditation and affirmations), you health will recover completely or, at least, partially.

Q   *What is considered low-carbohydrate (since there are so many theories that contradict)?*

A   Low-carbohydrate means that the carbohydrate gram count in a diet is low. Meats, fish, and dairy have little or no carbs. Nuts, fruit, vegetables, grains, some dairy and junk food contain carbs. Carbs assimilation and the blood sugar levels are balanced by insulin. During carbohydrate assimilation process you do not burn fat, and you can gain fat. Some protein diets say NO to carbs altogether; some say to eat less than 60 grams of carbs a day. Very-low-carbohydrate diets incorporate only 7 grams of carbs per meal. That amount of carbs has about the same effect on weight loss as does eating 0 grams, yet it gives you a bit of energy. At first, low-carbohydrate diets worked for me. Then my body learned the trick. My pancreas probably atrophied because it was never used, and I'd blow up with edema if I had one grape. Now I like my protein and carb balance to be almost equal. In the morning my carb/protein ratio is 70/30; in the afternoon—50/50; and in the evening—35/65. I like the energy from carbs in the morning.

Q   *What dieting principle holds true?*

A   The most important thing to remember is that whatever technique, method, trick or shortcut you used to lose your weight will be the very reason why it will back faster and more. You cut calories to lose weight? Then add a few more pounds for the few more calories you will add when go off the diet. You over-exercise to lose pounds? Then when you relax or return to normal exercise routine, your weight will creep back up.

Q   *Are tans healthy or harmful?*

A   Sunshine is a must. Not only for the Vitamin D, but sunshine is also a catalyst for other vitamins and minerals. It penetrates the pineal gland, through the eyes, which is great for thwarting depression and for increasing the release of serotonin. A slight tan or a little color is also a protective measure. It thickens the layers of melanin, which helps you not to burn from accidental sun overexposure. A burn will usually result if you expose white skin (with little melanin) to the sun for too long. The burn will not turn into a tan. It has to heal. If your burn turned to a tan, it was only because you peeled your burn off of the tan. Sunburns (not light suntans) will cause irreversible skin damage. Some fresh vegetables, like carrots, have carotene, which also adds color to your skin.

Q   *How much are addictive behaviors influenced by genes?*

A   Reportedly, genetic factors account for about 40% of the influence. But I believe that we can develop wisdom and learn from other people's "bottoming out." Rigorous honesty plays an important part because denial "blocks" our intuition, which drives us deeper into our disease. Yes, I have addiction in my genes. But I was lucky to have a strong spiritual family with a lot of recovery; their rigorous honesty and willingness to surrender helped me step onto the path of getting well.

Q   *How do brain chemicals affect addiction?*

A   It is rather complex and different for different people and at different times; but to put it simply, dopamine (a chemical in the brain that gives us a euphoric feeling) is released or sometimes over-released when we experience pleasure. In anticipation, the memory of such an experience also causes the release of dopamine, which causes cravings. Then from overindulging in this pleasure, we deplete dopamine, so we practice our addiction to restock at least some dopamine. This process does not enhance our pleasure, it just allows us not to crash. Other chemicals are released while we experience pleasure—such as serotonin, which is also depleted when overindulging in anything pleasurable. This, in simple terms, is the mechanism of addiction.

Q   *You talk about learned behavior. Explain that. How do you define "dysfunctional family?"*

A   Our parents or people who raise us are our involuntary role models in our childhood. Every family has problems or even skeletons in their closets. It is not the problems themselves, however, but how our role models deal with them that affects us. We are exposed to our caretakers' methods of dealing with or suppressing of these feelings. I observed drinking and eating being used as a stress release, social excuse, mood alternator and a necessity (when it was an addiction). However, my sis and I were also lucky to be surrounded by responsible, hard-working, honest, spiritual recovery in our family.

But in dysfunctional families, roles can reverse. We became the caretakers of the sick ones in our family. We fashioned strict boundaries for ourselves to follow. Normal kids follow guidelines, obey the rules and respect the limits taught to them by their parents. They also constantly engage in "testing" them. On the other hand, in a dysfunctional family, the kids are so full of fear of abandonment and shame from feeling that they are the problem, they do not rebel or test. Later, these kids, as we did, rebel for freedom or get addicted to rituals, patterns, rules and schedules to feel safe. It is a paradox, because it was hard for me to commit; yet I set a rigid discipline system to feel I was in control. I define a dysfunctional family as a family that has a drug/alcohol abuse, a major death or tragedy, severe religion (that emphasizes fear, guilt and shame), or secrets never discussed. What makes a dysfunctional family different from a normal one is the way it deals with these tragedies. Dysfunctional families usually suppress feelings, do not get recovery or pretend that things are fine. These suppressed feelings do not go away. In fact, they build up. And then they explode in a dysfunctional manifestation like rage, alcoholism, anorexia, etc. And it may work at first. But this temporary relief or escape does not make the problem go away, so the addict tries to get more relief from the addiction. Then the addiction becomes a bigger problem—and does not solve the old ones, either. Recovery means abstaining from the addiction so that our minds are clear, and recovery also means finding new healthy and honest ways of dealing with the original problems which are still there. I am not a victim from being in a dysfunctional family. On the contrary, I learned what does not work; I do not have to repeat those mistakes. And I observed what does work. This created an opening for me to find other choices and possibilities.

Q   *How can you call (for example) alcoholism or anorexia a disease? How does it compare to such "accepted" diseases, as cancer or diabetes?*

A   Most people say addictions are "chosen," unlike cancer or other physical maladies. But I've yet to see someone choose to be a drug addict or a compulsive overeater. Addicts do not choose pain or decide to lie, cheat and steal to practice their addiction. Addicts do not chose to have such hopelessness that they want to kill themselves (or do not care if they die). The addiction becomes the disease when it is destructive and life-threatening, even to the addict. When the body is sick and can't get well, the disease has taken the body over. When the brain is sick, it causes the body to get sick and the disease will kill, as in alcoholism or bulimia. However, addiction does not physically take over the body in a way cancer does; you can and must stop the symptom (drinking, using drugs, over- or under-eating) so that the brain is clear, and the body can regenerate. To keep you from returning to the "drug of choice," you need other healthy patterns so that there is no relapse. There's a chain of events that leads to sobriety or causes the return to addiction. It never just happens.

Q   *What is the difference between addiction and a strong desire?*

A   Simple. Desire is a strong urge that can be satisfied. It can turn into an addiction. Addiction is something that you can't live with or without. Sometimes there is no desire, just need. And you'll do it at any cost. We choose our desires. We do not choose our addictions.

Q *When you dated, what was the difference between a "normal" man and a man in full recovery? The same question about your female friends.*

A There is a difference, most definitely. Shane and I both prefer dates and friends with at least the desire for recovery. Recovery unfolds other aspects of your life that have to be cleaned up. It is a humbling experience to clean up, come clean and live clean. You see the profound wisdom in the eyes of someone who has been to Hell and back. It is an extra "X" factor that is alluring and attractive. I used to be a sucker for a masculine man, no matter how much of a degenerate he would be. Now I like to see strength and courage manifest in action. I do not go for men who act macho to conceal their deep-seated issues or fears. Chivalry to me is when a man is trustworthy and open—not into games and pretence. I like a man who is, yet not afraid to be spiritual and virtuous.

My girlfriends have similar qualities. I do not identify with superficial women who spend their lives learning to manipulate their bodies and men's brains in order to become the best gold-diggers. How sad it is that there are so many women who believe that their place in life is to spend half of their lives metamorphosing into "DIVA SEDUCTRESSES," and the other half—seducing the "men with the gold," whom they want to trap. Alas, our culture not only condones this but conditions young women to aspire to this.

Q *If you are working out or building muscle, which food group is more important: protein or carbohydrates?*

A There is no black-and-white answer. Protein is very important: it contains amino acids, the building blocks of our muscle tissue. It is important to incorporate high quality nitrogen-based foods (good protein sources like chicken breast, fish, eggs, nuts, etc.) in order to build good-quality muscle. Protein can sometimes serve as fuel, like carbohydrates. Carbs, on the other hand, cannot double as building blocks of our bodily tissues. Carbs are important for fuel as they constitute your "energy box."

You also need fat, which is a good source of energy. Fat (especially EFA oils) promotes the body's thermogenesis. Fat stimulates prostaglandis, "the cell's motors," essential for all living material.

Thus, I endorse all three food groups: protein, carbs, and fat—in balance. The carbs and protein should be eaten in about equal amounts, with about 15-25% of your total caloric intake to be in the form of fat. Having just a carbohydrate-containing snack before a workout may actually cause harm. If you eat a carb snack, add protein (or at least fat), or there may be an insulin overflow. When this happens, there is no "fat burning," so if your body needs fuel and can't find it, it may "steal" from your muscle reserves. A pure protein snack is insufficient for instant fuel. Protein also requires a lot of digestion, which will cause fatigue and dehydration. It is best to have a small, balanced snack like a piece of cheese and half an apple. Synergy is the key.

Q   *Should I only have egg whites? Can I eat yolks?*

A   Yolks contain certain ingredients (such as lecithin) that nature provided to break down and utilize the whites in the eggs properly. But be frugal. Yolks have cholesterol. Only add one or one-half of an egg yolk to two or three egg whites. Moderation and balance. I would stress the same with fruit. Juice and fructose are fragmented foods—not whole—the way nature intended. Fruit pulp helps slow down the insulin flow caused by fruit. Fragmented foods, such as juice, oxidize faster and are not recognized as a complete food by the body. Fiber also helps digestion. Once again, ingredients work synergistically, the way nature intended them to.

Q   *Why do more women than men fall victim to diets and other abusive measures?*

A   Well, the obvious reason (jokingly and for serious) is that men are attracted to pretty women; women are attracted to the "bulge" in the back pocket of a man. Unfortunately, a pretty girl, who follows those search criteria, never stays home on Friday or Saturday night, whereas a woman with a MENSA IQ and a nuclear physicist's degree might never "score." That's life!

Men would never put up with what women do—emotionally or physically. That's why women bear children. It is a proven fact that women can endure more pain than men can endure. So, women not only can, but also do end up going through insane diets to look good. In doing so, they ruin their metabolism. If men got a taste of their own medicine and were inundated with half-naked, perfect hard-bodied men, they would put up a stink. Yet, men count on women to put up with what men themselves would not. And women with a different outlook are branded jealous. I feel for the normal housewife trying to watch "family TV" with her spouse and kids, only to find out that the media caters to men. Is it not ridiculous that women (and gay men) exceedingly outnumber straight men, yet sexist TV, advertising, movies, etc., RULE!

Q   *How do you feel about young girls modeling, and about them being sometimes revered for their modeling?*

A   I think it is dangerous and unhealthy. Young minds are constantly molding, reinventing themselves and still searching. Modeling, unfortunately, is promoted in a sexual connotation. Once a young woman gets a "taste" of her power, sexually, it corrupts her and her young followers. Emphasis for young women should be on their education, their creative abilities, and the use of their bodies as vehicles for sports or contribution. Young ladies are easily influenced, so the younger the celebrity, the more of an impact she has. If a certain revered teenager makes a lot of money for looking good and being thin, that becomes her message to the millions who are in awe of her. If her focus is on her education in contrast to her body, and she uses modeling for experience and college funds, then this is more balanced. But we, as a society, put so much emphasis on beauty, sex and fame that those things seem to be the dominating message to our kids. It is a shame. But let's not be in denial or blame. We all have a voice!

Q   *Is it insecurity or the outside pressure that makes someone, especially a young person, anorexic or bulimic?*

A   It is a combination. It could be the lack of certain brain chemicals, such as serotonin, from a variety of reasons. Food addiction is also learned behavior, the use of "survival mechanisms" to deal with pain. Kids in dysfunctional families usually do not see that their role models are having a problem. The kids think they are the problem. Shame, guilt and fear makes it easy to for them to turn against themselves, to engage in destructive behavior. Then the solution becomes a bigger problem than the problem they are trying to suppress or escape.

Young children in dysfunctional families have contradicting feelings or live in a paradox. They do not have the normal boundaries or a "safe" atmosphere a "normy" child does. So they either "test" their limits or go too far (compulsive overeating or anorexia—starvation) because the "control" and freedom feels good. Or they feel safe in rituals, strict boundaries and unreasonable control as the "fix" for the situation. Young victims are unable to commit because they do not trust themselves, yet their rules and standards, which they force themselves to abide by, make them feel secure. It is truly a paradox, which <u>later</u> turns into insecurity and becomes subject to influence by the media pressure. But insecurity is <u>never</u> the reason! All adolescents feel pressure or insecurity while they are discovering themselves. Dysfunctional kids just deal with this pain more destructively.

Q   *Of all the ingredients for good health (exercise, diet, fresh air, sun and plenty of rest), which is the most important?*

A   If I were to stress one over the others, it would be <u>rest</u>. However, all of those elements relate to rest. Our job is not to "fix" the body; it is to minimize the amount of toxins and unnecessary processing, so we can let our sophisticated bodies do their job! The more we rest, the more the body rejuvenates, heals and regenerates itself. Proper exercise and fresh air provide the bodily tissues with the oxygen they need, which in turn helps the body rest and not overwork. A clean diet is easily assimilated and moves through our bodies more efficiently, producing the most benefits. Meaning, everything we do should be to embellish our needed rest. You can't cheat sleep. You obviously need less of it if you take better care of yourself. The body follows biorhythmic patterns. It digests, then eliminates, then heals. So, do not burden your body with unnecessary drugs or foods. Juice fasting and <u>rest</u> are the best remedies for most illnesses.

Q   *What makes some people stronger, thinner or healthier? Is it genes, discipline or luck?*

A   Genes and discipline—yes. No such thing as continuous good luck. Things flow in the direction we desire or will them to. What makes a body strong? Muscles. Muscles are only a manifestation of moving energy, dictated by our mind. Meaning, the mind is where the strength originates. We cultivate discipline through the mind to build the muscle. I think our genes give both our brains and our muscles the template of what we should or can be. If we eat right, exercise and practice good health routines—we groom our bodies like a soldier preparing for combat. Without mental affirmation, our genes do not produce good luck on their own. They can only give us a good kick-start. The best success stories I've heard came from Olympics trainees who were the underdogs with disadvantages or handicaps, who succeeded on pure will, determination and desire.

Q   *If something is labeled "organic," is it?*
A   Only if it reads "<u>certified</u>" organic.

Q   *When you exercise, what is the best food to eat for quick energy?*

A   True energy actually comes from the process called catabolism. Even a healthy protein and fruit snack, eaten shortly before the exercise, will actually only act as a stimulant by raising both the heartbeat and blood sugar. But more importantly, that snack will be used to build more tissue (this process is called anabolism), instead of providing us with the needed energy.

Q   *The word "co-dependent" seems to be an overused phrase.*

What exactly does it mean?

A   Well, it seems to be "hip" to be co-dependent, only because almost everyone is, and therapy is very fashionable. Co-dependency is an addition to people, places or things. Co-dependent literally means "dependent with". The alcoholic's spouse is not the only co-dependent. The alcoholic himself is co-dependent to his alcohol, in a sense. My personal definition of a co-dependent is "a person who thinks she is addiction-free, and who is just "helping" (controlling) the addict. The sickest co-dependent is as sick as a drug addict is, because she will stay in an unhealthy relationship to the point of destroying her own life, waiting for the other person to change.

Q   *Why do women crave sugar more than men?*

A   There is a solid body of research which finds that women have lower levels of serotonin (see definition in our glossary), which results in increased cravings for sugar (carbohydrates cause serotonin spikes—naturally). Certainly, this phenomenon, along with psychological pressure, causes a higher frequency of food disorders in women.

More scary diet stories

NOTE FROM THE EDITOR: Unlike the rest of the book, some of these stories are written by Shane Barbi—they are marked accordingly

Scary diet story 28

The very first diet we attempted was when we were in high school. We were far from being fat, even called thin by some. But it was fashionable to proclaim your diet of the week. We chose a protein diet since it allowed all the protein and fat we could eat. We felt like ranch hands. And it sure was fun eating as much as we could. To us, living on a ranch wasn't about "what" we were having for dinner, but "who" we were having for dinner. Tommy, Sara and Gigi were not dinner guests; they were our dinner entrees. That probably was what motivated us to become vegetarians. We did not lose weight on the protein diet. Besides, all we could think about was the sweet, succulent fruit that was forbidden—like Eve with the apple. So, we resolutely moooo-ved on to the next diet.

Scary diet story 29

After our second Playboy shoot and after being naked for two weeks, we were itching to put our clothes back on. We layered ourselves until we looked like Eskimos in the middle of winter. It looked a bit strange in the Caribbean. So, our next strategy was to be able to eat like wrestlers, but to keep our health-food and good-discipline reputation. It was tricky. We would follow what we called good twin/bad twin strategy. One of us would stay with our Playboy entourage, while the other would sneak away during our layover at the airport and stock up. Stocking up meant filling every empty carry-on accessory and every pocket. We would even pad our stomachs; we looked like pregnant women. The strategy was simple, except for one problem. My sister looked like the Unibomber. Shane wearing everything that had a pocket or room for food provided for strange look. Even her hat was a great place to store food. Shane's winter apparel, her hat and glasses—on a hot summer day in Puerto Rico— made her stick out like a drug lord. I saw my sister way in the yonder giving me a "thumbs up," which meant everything was going well. But she did not notice the security guards behind her, ready to stop and frisk her. I was way too embarrassed to save her. What's worse than one Unibomber? Two Unibombers who look exactly the same. So, I disloyally let her handle it on her own.

However, I thought she would not be able to make the plane ride home with our entourage, so I would have to stay and wait for her. Not because of sibling loyalty, but because of binge buddy loyalty. How could I binge without my buddy? Better yet, how could I binge without my foods that were about to be confiscated? No way. Nothing would ruin those plans. So, there I went, "Super-Sis" to the rescue.

Scary diet story 30 (by Shane Barbi)

Our mother told this story. At a very young age, my sister and I would carry backpacks or duffel bags everywhere we went. Our motive? To store food like hamsters. I guess we were like bears before hibernation. Whenever we went someplace, we were afraid of getting hungry, even though our mother faithfully made sure we had three square meals a day. We were filling a void, and if it didn't fit in our stomachs; our bag of the week would be our surrogate stomach. What I do not understand is why no one noticed it or stopped us. We'd come into a place "light-handed" and leave dragging what looked like a dead body. Maybe our skinny little bodies made us appear as though our mom was starving us.

Scary diet story 31 (by Shane Barbi)

We knew the right combinations of laxatives and the varieties to swallow in order to outsmart our body's recruiting system for fat. We would first mix organic natural cleansers before we ate. Then we would follow up with an intestinal roto-rooter as we ate. And finish off with a blast of dynamite after we ate. I'm sure the South American drug cartel would have been impressed with our laxative supply and demand. We would time our overdose from the "excuse me, I have to head for the ladies room," to the "I feel like I'm aborting, I'll never do this again!" only to reiterate the very same words the next day, adding a few more color combos to the variety-pack we invented. We were up to nearly 100 laxatives each a day. We were smart enough to stay home.

During one not-so-well-planned laxative session we accidentally took our laxatives at the same time, and too many of them. Who would be the nurse's aide? Well, lucky for me, I dropped first to the ground, while my sister's intestines were still intact, and her fingers could hit redial. There I was, on the floor, with a little froth flowing from my mouth. Not our typical calendar shot! My sis was able to do our usual "911" panic call to a doctor who specialized in poisons. We were lucky. This doctor was brilliant in his specialty. (How would I know? I was busy with other things; I just took her word.) She helped me recover (with his assistance). No sooner than when I was about to thank the doctor, my sister dropped to the floor—almost in my exact chalk outline—with the same symptoms of froth oozing, etc. etc. At first, I thought she was imitating me. How rude! But the froth looked so real. Oh, dear, by this time she was in no position (no pun intended) to outline the instructions given to her for me.

So, I simply pressed redial on the phone so I could talk to the same doctor. "No, no, no, this is her sister," I embarrassingly argued—the doctor did not think it was possible that the exact same thing could happen again—with a familiar voice asking for help. He inquired, "Wow, are you two twins?" I said, "Huh?" as I sweated profusely. He repeated, "Twins, you know, like the Barbi Twins?" Busted! (No pun again). I then spent a well invested twenty minutes explaining how different my older, much larger, much tanner sister and I were in all ways. Not only we weren't twins, we were stepsisters, and not alike in any way! Our voices only coincidentally sounded alike because we had both happened to overdose on laxatives at the same time. What a hoot that he would think that two such opposite looking people could be twins! While my long-winded alibi presentation continued, my poor neglected sis crawled into the bathroom like a wounded animal finding a place to die.

When she finally recovered, she was so mad that I had the nerve to lie to the doctor about us. She could not believe I'd be more concerned about saving our reputation than about her intestines doing somersaults! Boy, did she have a sweet revenge in mind for me to teach me a lesson. She told me she was going to send the sweet doctor an autographed laxative box and sign it, "Thank you! Love, Barbi Twins."

Scary diet story 32

Don't you think that those misleading food photos on covers of diet packages should be outlawed? I know they are award-winning photos of dishes by a famous French chef, but they just don't correlate with the astronaut food (circa 1968), sealed inside. The taste of those doll-food meals is more like the cardboard box they come in. How dare they make diet cookies or candies so small and tasteless! Dieting is bad enough!

I guess every dieter looks for the magical food that tastes great but has absolutely no calories or fat. And why can we put men on the moon, cure disease and create smart bombs, and not be able to invent tasty, no-calorie, no-fat desserts? Well, we did.

We went to every health food store and bought everything from gelatin to sweeteners to pectin; anything labeled "No fat" or "no calories." This was dreamy—until we baked this Frankenstein nightmare. Although it smelled good, it looked more like a Stephen King character. We then wrapped it in tinfoil. Everything seems to taste like Mom's homemade pie when it is wrapped in tinfoil. We were planning to save it for a reward snack in New York, between jobs. In case this new invention did a "Nutty Professor" reversal on us, we would not try it until we finished work.

We needed lab rats to sample our formula. We knew that people that worked for us were co-dependent enough not to say no. One employee sampled our snack. "I dropped it on my toe and it broke! My toe. The snack stayed perfectly intact," he revealed. We could not understand his attitude—when we finally got to eat our tasty delight, we loved it. It was delicious. If he had fasted for a day or two, he would not be so finicky. Remember, as the saying goes, gratefulness is the road to recovery. Or were our taste buds in denial?

Scary diet story (33 by Shane Barbi)

Growing up on a ranch was hard work. The hard part was working with all that food: food we grew, food we made food that was alive and food we cooked. Life was about food when you lived on a ranch, and when you didn't work, you were eating. When you finally got to sit down and eat the food, you wanted to take your time; a lot of time meant a lot more food to eat. The choice was either to rest and eat one more piece of pie, or to go back to work. Guess what choice I made? (Hint: I had about four more pieces of pie.)

My favorite chore was gathering the fruit and vegetables from the "South Forty" on our ranch. The strawberries tasted like they were dipped in a sweetener, and the carrots—as though they were covered with melted butter. One day, on a beautiful, sunny afternoon, I went out to gather the crop. For some reason, the fruit and vegetables looked especially good—gleaming in the sunlight—like those plastic, expensive fruit baskets, which you see in department stores. I wanted to nibble in the "pasture," imitating the animals on the ranch. It must have been quite a sight to see me grazing in the yonder. The problem was, I had already eaten lunch and this was my "assigned" chore: to gather the crop (not to graze on it) and to bring it home. I do not know if I had a long-winded imagination or just a long-winded food disorder, but it seemed that I ate up the whole

South Forty. I prayed for an earthquake, fire, or flood to camouflage my "wipe-out". No such luck. Needless to say, my next assigned chore was to work with animals only … live animals.

At about the same time, my sister was in Hawaii. (We were separated most of our lives, but shared our food problem no matter what the geographical distance between us was.) I called my sister in Hawaii to report on my newly assigned chore. Her neighbor had to retrieve her from a fruit tree of her choice, in her front yard. It was easy spotting the tree of the day. Sis's legs were dangling frantically from the mango tree. Now I know why her teeth were shorter than normal. All that fruit acid took its toll on her teeth. I knew not to disturb her in the middle of her grazing, so I just left a message with her neighbor.

Scary diet story 34 (by Shane Barbi)

Photo shoots have taken us to countless beautiful tropical resorts. One time in particular stands out in our minds because of our insane behavior. We felt very insecure and needed to eat in order to decide if we wanted to finish the shoot. We needed that glycogen in the brain to think, and it comes in many beautiful forms: tropical fruit dipped in chocolate, fancy pastries, fattening meals. So, feeling a bit of shame, we paid off a restaurant to let us in after hours. We didn't bother with meals. We had them roll over the dessert tray (6 levels), and we tried every piece of culinary art. As soon as we got sane from eating the food, we realized we didn't have a choice—we had a contract to finish the shoot and had only 13 hours to be restored to normal size. We had a busy night of bathroom aerobics. As long as our stomachs were flat, we could care less about the bags under our eyes—they could always be "airbrushed" out. I recall the retouchers saying, "We could only airbrush so much of the bags and red eyes!"

Scary diet story 35

One of our healthier diet experiences was when we were hygienic—that meant eating raw foods—no meat—in perfect combinations. In other words, we were fanatical and not practical. We got high on being healthier than most people (part of the perfectionism of the disease.) We were the type who, after reading about certain saints, would also want to eat just a communion wafer a day. Not because we tried to be spiritual, but so that God might help us starve. At the time, we did not consider "fat farms" to be spiritual. So we hit hygienic institutions that specialized in fasting. Now we could starve in the name of health, with the help of God, owing to the spiritual literature we brought with us to read. This was a slam-dunk. We made several attempts and failed several times. One time we actually completed twenty days of water fasting.

Mostly, our fasts were interrupted with orgasmic binges reenacted like the "greatest escape from Alcatraz." The planning of these great escapes made the drool in our mouths tastier than eating the actual evidence at the scene of the crime. The hygienic institution was located in the middle of nowhere; I'm sure, for a good reason. My sis and I schemed like Dream Team lawyers, negotiating good excuses to break our fast and live out our desires—one last time.

We caught a ride to town with some young local driving a truck full of oranges. We sat in the back with the oranges. With the lawyer mentality working our brains, we justified snacking as the means to prepare our stomachs for the Roman feast we were hoping to encounter at the nearest place that resembled a 7-11. Our ride lasted about one and a half hours. So did our snack. We should have received some kind of an award for the artwork of making 200 oranges in 10 box crates look completely untouched. By this time, our stomachs were way too stuffed, and our teeth and gums were way too sore, to enjoy the entrée of our life that had awaited us at 7-11. What a torture! Oh, well, back to the drawing board to plan our next escape and "food-free" ride (as compared to a free-food ride.)

Scary diet story 36 (by Shane Barbi)

Most of our lives, we have been very thin. Even when we thought we were obese, we were far from that point. But our extreme feast-to-famine diet habits manifested strange physical appearances. During fasts, our eyes would sink, and our fingers would look like bony witch claws. During binges, I'd bloat, sometimes in just one area, like my feet and ankles, especially on a plane. After laxatives I'd be frightfully dehydrated and sometimes bruised under the eyes. After purging, my fingers would be pruney, and I'd have bad breath and puffy red eyes. All of this just to look GOOD? You see, thin = beauty! My sister and I never noticed or cared about such "trivial" side effects as a heart attack.

We should not have been responsible for picking out some of our pictures for magazines. We would choose a picture, which made us look thinner, no matter how scary our faces looked. If someone said, "In this picture you look like the Night of the Living Dead," that was our pick of the week to be printed for millions! (Distorted thinking and vision!) If someone said, "You girls look pretty and healthy here," into the paper shredder it would go.

The most embarrassing memorable moment was after a twenty-day fast on water. I wanted to binge after, thinking I deserved it and it would not show. At first, I got full in the stomach but not in the brain. I wanted to eat every food that was mentioned during my fast: food seen on TV, food I saw in a magazine, food I smelled at neighbors' homes, and food I fantasized about while trying to sleep at night during my fast. It took about three days before I finally ate about half of my desired goodies without showing any weight gain. I only planned on one binge day, but I felt ripped off not "living out" my desires before I had to go back to a boring diet to maintain my thin body.

Well, on the fourth day, I had almost completed my forbidden taboo thirst for my goodies. As I was waddling out of the health food store to get into my car, I had to unsnap and slightly unzip my jeans. My stomach really hurt. I was constipated from the shock of eating all that food after a fast, and gas was trying to build up if there was enough room in my intestines because they were swollen from being overworked. Thank God I wore a long, loose "tent" for a shirt. A woman came running towards me with the biggest, zealous smile. She put her hands on my stomach and enthusiastically asked me, "How many months are you?" My life flashed in front of me. Sure, I still had my skinny limbs, neck and frame, but my STOMACH had started to rebel. It was crying for help and I ignored it like a neglected child.

I was red with humiliation. But being co-dependent as well, how could I tell her that I had gas build-up, had been pigging out for four days, and I had been practicing my celibacy for the last six months!" It was easier to say, "Oh, about four months, almost five." (That would make it an Immaculate Conception.) She then replied, "Boy, you hardly show for four and a half months, you're lucky!" I had the nerve (and distorted thinking) to thank her and feel good about nourishing my infant. Suddenly, I had the urge for pickles and ice cream!

Scary diet story 37

Our experience with laxatives made astute pharmacists of us. We learned the perfect combinations, perfect timing, and had the phone set on redial at 911 in case anything went wrong. We would carefully time ourselves; one of us would be the guinea pig, the other a nurse. We knew the laxatives had stopped working altogether when the only thing evacuating from my body was froth from my mouth. I was in critical condition, but refused to go to the hospital. I didn't want to end up with a gravestone that read, "defecated to death." The doctor warned me, "If you do this one more time, you could die." I could have sworn he said, "You have one more time."

The Barbis' glossary

These simple straightforward definitions are relevant to the context of this book. The glossary contains only limited information, but may be helpful in understanding many of the terms used throughout.

Acid—A substance that release hydrogen ions. Acidosis is an increase in hydrogen ions and a major cause of exercise fatigue. Acids can be either organic or inorganic compounds.

Acidophilus—Beneficial live bacteria essential for healthy intestinal function.

Acidosis—a blood condition in which the bicarbonate concentration is below normal; often produced by fermentation of proteins and carbohydrates because mineral salts are not present in food.

Acute illness—A sickness that comes on quickly and may cause severe symptoms, but is of short duration.

Adaptogen—The term for a substance that produces suitable adjustments in the body. Some beneficial adaptogens include garlic, ginseng, echinacea, gingko biloba and goldenseal.

Adrenal glands—Glands situated on top of the kidneys that secrete different types of hormones.

Aerobic—With oxygen. Aerobic exercise utilizes oxygen in the fuel burning process; it encompasses any type of sustained and rhythmic movement. The main fuels for aerobic energy are carbohydrates and fats.

AIDS—Acquired immune deficiency syndrome.

Aloe Vera—A juice or jell-like substance derived from Aloe plant; prevents scarring from wounds, burns and abrasions. Aloe juice is sometimes used for digestion and as a natural laxative.

Allergen—A substance that provokes an allergic response.

Allergy—An inappropriate defensive response by the immune system to a normally harmless substance.

Amino acid—The building blocks of proteins; any of 22 nitrogen-containing organic acids essential for synthesizing proteins in your body.

Anaerobic—With little or no oxygen. Anaerobic exercise utilizes a limited amount of oxygen in the fuel burning process, as in stop-and-go activities like weight lifting and wind sprints. In these activities, glycogen is immediately available to muscles and the liver for short bursts of exercise.

Anemia—A hemoglobin deficiency in blood which affects its ability to carry oxygen to the bodily tissues.

Antacid—A substance that neutralizes acid in the stomach.

Antibody—A protein molecule that neutralizes a specific invading organism in the body.

Antioxidant—A protective substance that inhibits destructive oxidation reactions at the cellular level. Examples include vitamins C and E, the minerals selenium and germanium, some amino acids, etc.

Astragalus root—Astragalus membranaceus. An herb that helps fight extreme fatigue and aids immune system.

Autoimmune disorder—A condition in which the body's immune system rejects and attacks the body's own tissues. Examples include multiple sclerosis, rheumatoid arthritis, systemic lupus erythematosus, etc.

Autolysis—A process, whereby the bodily tissue is broken down by the action of enzymes contained in the tissue affected; self-digestion. Body literally feeds on itself breaking down less important tissue to feed vital tissue. Like a potato in water growing roots—this is the same process in fasting, during ketosis.

Bacteria—Single-celled microorganisms. Harmful bacteria can cause disease; friendly bacteria aid digestion, protect the body, and engage in other vital functions.

Bee pollen—A natural substance collected by bees from male seed flowers, mixed with secretions from the bee and molded into granules. Bee pollen is high in vital nutrients and amino acids; can be used to combat allergies.

Bee propolis—A product collected by bees from the resin under the bark of certain trees. It is an antibiotic substance that boosts immunity and fights infection.

Benign—Considered harmless or not cancerous.

Bentonite—A natural clay substance used for elimination of the body's toxins and bacteria.

Beta-carotene—The chemical precursor to vitamin A; an antioxidant.

Bile—A compound made in the liver, stored in the gall bladder and secreted in the small intestine, when needed. It readies fats and oils for digestion. Bile is alkaline; it acts to counteract acidity in the stomach.

Bioflavonoids—Plant compounds found in citrus fruit and green leafy vegetables. Known collectively as vitamin P, they exhibit antioxidant properties and are sometimes prescribed for allergies and inflammations as it acts to strengthen cellular membranes by maintain the resistance of capillary walls to permeation and change of pressure.

Boron—A trace mineral found in legumes and some fruit; may help prevent bone loss and arthritis. Beneficial for bone and muscle building.

Bran—The outside shell of the grain with the highest form of fiber content; helps digestion, elimination and other health functions.

Brewer's yeast—A rich source of protein, B vitamins, amino acids and minerals, such as chromium. Helps steady blood sugar and metabolism, reduce serum cholesterol and raise levels of HDLs. It also aids healing by producing large amounts of collagen; improves skin texture and blemishes. Intake of Brewer's yeast should be avoided during yeast infections.

Bromelain—A natural enzyme, found in pineapple, that aids metabolism and energy, relieves muscle pain and swelling and promotes wound healing. Found in wine and cheese.

Broom foods—High-fiber, wholesome foods including bran, grains, fruit and vegetables.

Canola oil—The oil from the rapeseed plant; high in monounsaturated fat.
Capillaries—Tiny blood vessels that allow the exchange of nutrients and wastes between the bloodstream and cells.
Capsium—A catalyst which synergistically enhances other herbs. Promotes thermogenesis, aiding weight loss and increasing circulation.
Carbohydrate—An organic substance—almost always of plant origin—the major source of energy in the diet.
Carcinogen—A substance that may cause cancer.
Carob powder—Natural, sweet powdered sugar similar to chocolate, but contains less fat and no caffeine.
Carotene—A yellow to orange pigment that is converted into vitamin A in the body.
Cell—A small, complex organic unit consisting of a nucleus, cytoplasm and a cell membrane. All living tissues are composed of cells.
Cerebral—Pertaining to the brain.
Charcoal— A safe, nontoxic agent that relieves gas and diarrhea, and many digestive disturbances.
Chelated—Bound to an amino acid for better absorption. When attached to minerals, it enables better assimilation. Remember, if your minerals are not ionic, they are merely crushed rocks. Every trick helps assimilation.
Chiropractic—A system of healing based on the belief that disorders and imbalances generally result from misalignments of the vertebrae.
Chitosan—A marine fiber concentrate that adheres to and binds lipids in the stomach causing fat and weight reduction.
Chlorella—A single-cell algae plant, rich with protein, fiber, beta-carotene and other high-quality nutrients. Boosts energy and the immune system.
Chlorophyll—The green color of plant tissues; essential to the production of carbohydrates by photosynthesis. Chlorophyll-rich products can be taken raw as diet supplements.
Cholesterol—A sterol which naturally occurs in bodily tissues. A necessary constituent of cell membranes for the transport and absorption of fatty acids. Excess cholesterol is a threat to health. Yet insufficient cholesterol is dangerous, as well. Healthy normal cholesterol levels range between 180 to 200 mg/dl.
Chromium—An essential trace mineral found in brewer's yeast, organ meats, whole grains and cheese. In the body, chromium helps stabilize insulin production, thus causing weight reduction. Chromium also helps even out blood sugar and reduce blood fat content and cholesterol.
Chromium picolinate—The combination of chromium and picolinic acid, a natural substance secreted by the liver and kidneys. Chromium helps level the body's insulin. Controversial studies show that it may build muscle, promote growth and help healing.
Chronic illness—A disorder that persists for a long duration, such as hay fever or diabetes.
Citric acid—An organic acid found in citrus fruit. Helps pH balance.
Co-enzyme—A molecule that works with an enzyme to enable it to perform its specific function. Co-enzymes are necessary in the utilization of vitamins and minerals.

Co-enzyme Q10—A vitamin-like antioxidant compound that helps fight heart disease and high blood pressure, improve athletic performance and boost immunity.

Colic—A malfunction of the digestive system, involving abdominal pain, distension and a painful intestinal spasm.

Colloids—A suspension composed of a continuous medium throughout which are dispersed small particles, 1 to 1000 nm in size, as opposed to crystalloids, particles smaller than colloids which are capable of forming a true solution. Colloids can pass through semipermeable membranes; crystalloids can not. Our body is able to digest and recognize colloids, as opposed to crystalloids, which, due to their ability to rush through our digestive tract, are not absorbed (unless chelated, etc, etc.). Certain supplements, such as free-form amino acids, minerals, etc, unless in food, will mostly not be absorbed.

Complex carbohydrate—A type of carbohydrate comprised of long-stringed molecules; it is converted into blood glucose slowly. Sources of complex carbohydrates also contain fiber. Good sources of complex carbohydrates include whole grains and wheat cereals.

Creatine—an amino acid that is a constituent of the muscles of vertebrates. Naturally occurring in meat; when taken as a supplement, it increases muscular cell water retention, allowing increased energy for muscular contraction, thus facilitating muscle gain.

Cross-linkage—Refers to the phenomenon of amino acid linking. Sun damage causes cross-linkage in our skin. Overcooking of food causes cross-linkage, thereby reducing assimilation and usability of the food.

Cruciferous—A term used to refer to a group of vegetables including broccoli, Brussels sprouts, cabbage, cauliflower and turnips, which have cross-shaped blossoms. These vegetables may help prevent colon cancer.

Dementia—A permanent acquired impairment of intellectual function.

Dermis—The layer of skin that lies underneath the epidermis.

Detoxification—The act of reducing the buildup of poisonous substances.

DHEA—dehydroepiandrosterone: a steroidal hormone produced in the adrenal glands (a precursor of testosterone). Its synthetic form is used as a nutritional supplement used to cause increase in lean muscular mass. Best if taken when you are over 40 years of age.

Diabetes—A disease that occurs when the pancreas fails to produce adequate insulin. Symptoms are mental confusion, coma, blindness and poor circulation.

Diet—A food plan that restricts calorie consumption, often to 1,000 calories or below, and does not incorporate balanced nutrition principles.

DiMethil—Glycine—(B15) a tissue oxygenator; used by athletes for top endurance.

DNA—Deoxyribonucleic acid. A substance in the cell nucleus that contains the cell's genetic blueprint and determines the type of life form into which a cell will develop.

Dulse—A sea vegetable used as a salt substitute or as diet tea.

Edema—Water retention, a condition that causes the body to bloat from spilled cellular fluids. A common response of the lymphatic system—body's way of searching for protein, normally occurring during dieting or fasting. Since protein can not be stored in the body, during fasting, lymphatic system searches for available protein, robbing bodily tissues. Sometimes, even when not dieting, one can still bloat. It is due to the fact that the body is then searching for extra protein to build antibodies to combat infection. Eating protein produces a dehydrating effect.

EDTA—Ethylene-diamine-tetra-acetic acid. An amino acid that fights free radicals and enhances minerals.

EEG—Electroencephalogram. A graph used to measure brain activity.

EKG—or EKG)-Electrocardiogram. A graph that monitors and measures heart function.

Eicosanoids—A form of fatty acids found primarily in fish oils— mini hormones within our cells which help dictate every action in the body. Good eicosanoids can reduce inflammation, strengthen immune system and lower blood fat and cholesterol. Taken in excess, they can reduce the blood clotting capability.. Bad Eicosanoids contribute to pain, bleeding etc. Aspirin is a blocker of bad eicosanoids. Essential fatty acids are the building blocks of eicosanoids. Linoleic acid is the only truly essential fat.

Electrolytes—Vital mineral compounds that maintain the body's fluid balance; they are capable of conducting electrical impulses.

Emulsion—A mix two of liquids that do not mix with each other, such as oil and water. Emulsification is the first step in the digestion of fat.

Endocrine system—The system of glands that secrete hormones. Endocrine glands include the pituitary, thyroid, thymus, and adrenal glands, the pancreas, ovaries and testes.

Endorphin—"Feel-good" chemicals released in the brain (i.e.; a runner's high). These natural opiates increase tolerance to pain and create feelings of well-being.

Enzymes—Protein catalysts that initiate or speed chemical reactions in the body.

Epidermis—The outer layer of skin.

Essential—A necessary nutrient; not manufactured by the body and must be supplied in the diet.

Essential fatty acids—Linoleic acid, linolenic acid, arachidonic acid —major components of all cell membranes. They help energy production and endocrine system function, regulate hormone and metabolic functions, ease PMS and menopause symptoms, and more.

Ester C—is a buffered version of vitamin C, from a natural source. This form of vitamin C stays in the body longer since vitamin C is water-soluble, and Ester C is not.

Estrogen—A female reproductive hormone, produced primarily in the ovarian follicles and stored in fat. The more fat you eat, the more estrogen you store. A high-fiber, lowfat diet drops the level of estrogen in the body; a too-high level is associated with PMS, irregular periods, uterine fibroids, breast and ovarian cancers and a late (or dangerous) menopause. This hormone is naturally occurring in seeds, vitamin E, wheat germ, dong quai, yams, etc. If your have fibroids, reduce these foods, especially caffeine. Too much vitamin C, citrus or even carbohydrates also mimic estrogen, and destroys your B vitamins, which causes a hormonal imbalance. Tofu and other soybean products contain phytoestrogens (plant estrogen) which help regulate estrogen levels in the body.

Fat-soluble—Capable of dissolving in fat and oils.

Fatty acids—Organic acids from which fat and oils are made.

Fiber—The indigestible portion of plant matter. It is capable of binding to toxins and escorting them out of the body.

Flaxseed oil—High in omega 3, an excellent source of unsaturated fatty acids.

Fo-Ti—A flavonoid rich herb used for energy and circulation.

Free radical—An atom or group of atoms that has at least one unpaired electron. Free radicals can attack cells and cause body damage.

Fructose—A simple fruit sugar.

Fungus—A class of organisms that includes yeasts, mold and mushrooms. Some are capable of causing severe disease.

Gamma Linoleic Acid (GLA)—Naturally occurs in primrose oil, borage oil or black currant oil. A source of energy; helps regulate hormonal balance and metabolism.

Gamma Oryzanol—a substance naturally occurring in rice bran oil, which has hormonal and vitamin—like effects on sex organs.

Garcinia Cambogia—is an Indian fruit used as a curry ingredient. It also contains active ingredients, which aid weight reduction.

Garlic—Therapeutic food with antioxidant properties that stimulates the liver to identify toxins and fight disease and infection.

Germanium—A trace mineral, excellent for immune system and energy.

Ginger—A spicy herb that has health properties, which aid digestion, alleviate headaches and other conditions.

Ginkgo biloba—A leaf or leaf extract; fights aging process, improves circulation, increases memory and has antioxidant properties.

Ginseng—A tonic herb that provides energy, helps stress and fatigue, builds endurance. Stimulates brain activity, aids memory, enhances male reproductive and circulatory systems.

Gland—An organ or tissue that secretes a substance for use elsewhere in the body rather than for its own functioning.

Globulin—Protein found in the blood, which contains disease-fighting antibodies.

Gluconeogenesis—Glucose formation in the body from a non-carbohydrate source, as from protein or fats. During fasting, this process starts when the body is done with ketosis. Gluconeogenesis usually starts after 21 days of fasting. Unlike in ketosis, during gluconeogenesis the body does not directly use fat for energy, it first converts fat, or protein into glucose, thus destroying important organic tissue.

Glucose—A simple sugar, present in blood as blood sugar, is the main source of energy for the body's cells.

Gluten—Protein found in many grains.

Glycemic Index—The relative potency of carbohydrates and their propensity to raise and stabilize blood sugar. (Recent research shows that are advantages to consuming lower glycemic foods, i.e., lentils, rather than high glycemic foods, i.e. potatoes, for use in exercise and athletic function.)

Glycerin—A naturally occurring carbohydrate-like substance found in coconuts. Used in natural cosmetics as a smoothing agent.

Glycogen—A tasteless polysaccharide, which serves as the principal carbohydrate, used by the body for energy — stored in the liver and muscles.

Gotu Kola—A caffeine-free stimulant herb. Helps restore energy; aids healing.

Green Tea—Has powerful antioxidant and anti-allergenic properties, used mostly for energy and clear thinking. Rich in flavonoids.

Guarana—A rainforest shrub from South America. Contains natural caffeine and guaranine, which give long-lasting energy without the highs-and-lows or the bad of hydrocarbons found in coffee.

Hemoglobin—An iron-containing red pigment in the blood responsible for the transport of oxygen.

HIV—Human immunodeficiency virus—the virus that causes AIDS.

Homeopathy—A medical methodology based on the belief that taking a minute dose of a substance, that would produce symptoms like those being treated, can cure illness. Small amount of certain drugs derived from the disease itself.

Honey—A sweet, viscous fluid produced by bees from the flower nectar and stored in nests or hives, used as a natural raw sweetener, twice as sweet as sugar. May have antibiotic and antiseptic properties; contains vitamins and enzymes.

Hormones—Essential substances produced by the endocrine glands that regulate many bodily functions.

Human Growth Hormone—Somatotropin, a polypeptide hormone secreted by the pituitary gland, that promotes growth before puberty, and after puberty, keeps the body in the muscle building, fat burning process. Growth Hormone can also increase your bone mass. Inhibitors are insulin and aging process. Growth Hormone release is enhanced by sleep, protein intake, fasting and anaerobic exercise.

Hydrochloric acid—An inorganic acid produced in the stomach to aid in digestion.

Hydrogenation—The amount of hydrogen atoms involved in chemical processes of fatty acid molecules.

Hypoallergenic—Having low capacity for inducing allergic reactions.

Hypoglycemia—Low blood sugar. Symptoms include fatigue and weakness, headache and irritability; panic attacks and anger.

Hypotension—Low blood pressure.

Hypothalamus—A portion of the brain that helps regulates metabolic activities, including body temperature and the hunger response.

Immune system—A constitution of functions and processes constituted by the interaction of many different organs, cells, hormones and proteins. Its chief function is to identify and eliminate foreign substances, such as harmful bacteria.

Immunity—The ability to resist disease or infection.

Infection—An invasion of bodily tissues by disease-causing organisms such as viruses, fungi or bacteria.

Insomnia—The inability to sleep.

Insulin—A hormone secreted by the pancreas that regulates the metabolism of glucose (sugar) in the body. Insulin allows cells to absorb and utilize glucose, stimulates glucose uptake by the liver and muscle and converts excess into fat storage. Exercise helps lower the amount of insulin needed to function optimally. An over-release of insulin is usually the basis of any weight problem and disease. Therefore, a properly balanced ratio of protein/fat/carbs can help insure continuous insulin balance, without causing an over-release.

Intestinal flora—"Friendly" bacteria in the intestines, essential for digestion.

IU—International unit reserved for some vitamins and minerals. A measure of potency based on an accepted international standard.

Kava—a Polynesian shrub, *Piper methysticum*, of the pepper family. When taken as an herbal supplement, in acts as a relaxant and mood enhancer.

Ketosis—The act of burning fat without burning glucose, which changes the acid/alkaline pH balance of your blood and can ultimately lead to coma and death. Usually occurs in diabetics who lack insulin to metabolize carbs, but can also affect strict dieters who consume insufficient and dangerously low levels of carbohydrates. Telltale signs include foul-smelling breath and urine.

Kola Nut—A seed from a tropical tree. A natural and rich source of caffeine and theobromine. Has stimulant effects without the highs-and-lows of coffee which contains hydrocarbons.

L-Carnitine—An amino acid that aids fat metabolism.

L-Tryptophan—An amino acid that stimulates serotonin and may ease depression and insomnia.

Lactase—An enzyme that converts lactose into glucose, necessary for the digestion of milk and milk products.

Lactic acid—Acid that results from anaerobic glucose metabolism. Present in certain foods, including certain fruit and sour milk. Also produced in the muscles during exercise; buildup of lactic acid in the body causes muscle fatigue.

Lactose Intolerance—Inability to break down and digest milk. Lactose is a substance found in milk and milk products. Inadequate production of lactase (see our enzyme section) in the small intestine results in the body's inability to digest lactose. Lactose intolerance is rare (but dangerous) in children, but common in adults, as with age, body's ability to digest lactose (milk sugar) lessens. Drinking milk after infancy results in improved lactose tolerance.

Lecithin—Fatty acid found in egg yolks and soybean products, which protects against heart disease, lowers cholesterol and boosts memory. Sometimes considered one of the B vitamins.

Lipid—A chemical family name for fats and related compounds, including choline, gamma-linolenic acid, inositol, lecithin and linoleic acid.

Lipoprotein—A protein molecule that incorporates a lipid. Lipoproteins act as agents of lipid transport in the lymph system and blood.

Lymphatic system (and lymph nodes)—a system of vessels and nodes transporting lymph, a clear coaguable fluid, resembling blood plasma, containing white blood cells. The lymphatic system moves nutrients (oxygen, nutrients, etc) to cells and transports cell waste and cell poisons away from tissues. This process doubles as the body's vital sewer system. Nodes are organs located in the lymphatic vessels that act as filters removing toxic and foreign material.

Macrobiotics—A diet based on eastern philosophy, focused on balancing the yin and yang energies of foods. The macrobiotic diet incorporates whole grain cereals, millet, rice and vegetables with beans, etc.

Malabsorption—The body's inability to absorb nutrients from the intestinal tract.

Melatonin—A hormone secreted by the pineal gland, which secretion is affected by the amount of light received by the retina. Taken as a supplement, it naturally enhances sleep and eases falling asleep.

Metabolism—Physical and chemical processes necessary to sustain life, including the production of cellular energy and synthesis of biological substances.

Microgram—A measurement of weight, equivalent to 1/1,000,000 of a gram.

Milligram—Measurement of weight equivalent to 1/1,000 of a gram. (A gram is equal to approximately 1/28 of an ounce.)

Minerals—Naturally occurring inorganic substances present in plants and animals essential for human life.

Miso—A fermented soybean paste, a therapeutic food that fights free radicals, helps the immune system and lowers cholesterol. Miso is a base for soups, sauces, dressings, dips, spreads and cooking stock and is a healthy substitute for salt.

Mitochondrion—A cellular power source, controlling cell metabolism and generating energy from energy sources, such as fat.

Molasses—An unsulphured by-product of sugar refinement, with high mineral content. Good for hair growth and natural hair color.

Neurotransmitters—Brain chemicals that transmit nerve impulses, i.e.: acetylcholine and dopamine.

Nucleic acids—A class of chemical compounds found in all viruses and plant and animal cells. Examples: RNA and DNA.

Nutrient—A substance that is needed by the body to maintain life and health.

Oats and oat bran—Beneficial grain and fiber sources that lower cholesterol and aid digestion and excretion. Oats are excellent as a long-term metabolic stimulant which, in its purest form, has been known to help addictions.

Octacosanol—wheat germ derivative — excellent for energy.

Oils, natural vegetable—Natural oils that contain vitamins and essential fatty acids.

Omega 3 oils—Essential fatty acids that prevent blood clotting, high cholesterol and high triglyceride levels. They improve stamina and hasten metabolism.

Organic—Foods that are grown without synthetic chemicals such as pesticides and hormones.

Oxalic acid—A white, water-soluble, poisonous acid; found in such foods as spinach, sodas, coffee, cocoa, chocolate, etc., that rob the body of nutrients, especially calcium.

Oxidation—A chemical reaction in which oxygen reacts with another substance, resulting in a chemical transformation. Oxidation of bodily tissues results in deterioration or spoilage.

pH—Potential of hydrogen. A scale used to measure acidity or alkalinity of substances. A pH of 7 is considered neutral; numbers below 7 show increasing acidity; numbers above 7 show increasing alkalinity. Too much alkalinity is from too much carbon dioxide (hyperventilating). The alkaline-acid ratio in the blood is normally 7.4 pH. Since the body cannot tolerate excess acids from the diet, it robs alkali in the body to neutralize excess acidity. Bodily pH is maintained in the kidneys (by the process of throwing off hydrogen ions from acids in the urine). Lungs excrete carbon dioxide (carbonate acid). Skin excretes hydrogen ions through sweating.

Pectin—A colloidal carbohydrate of high molecular weight; occurs in ripe fruit, especially in apples. Pectin helps with constipation.

Pituitary—A gland located at the base of the brain that secretes hormones regulating growth and metabolism.

Prostaglandin—A class of hormone-like chemical that are made in the body from essential fatty acids and have important effects on organs. They influence the secretion of hormones and enzymes, regulate an inflammatory response, blood pressure and blood clotting.

Protein—A class of complex nitrogen-based organic compounds constituted by different amino acids. Protein is the basic elements of all animal and vegetable tissue, and lack of sufficient protein can cause edema, muscle atrophy and even worse. Excess protein has a dehydrating effect on the body, and it leeches nutrients.

Psyllium husks—Fibrous seed husks from plants; they promote intestinal function, elimination, decrease appetite and suppress swings in blood sugar.

Pycnogenol—a strong bioflavonoid extract containing powerful antioxidant and memory enhancing capabilities.

Pyruvate—A naturally occurring substance which is important for energy metabolism. It is a bi-product of carb and fat metabolism.

RDA—Recommended daily allowance. The amount of a vitamin or other nutrient that should be consumed daily in order to prevent nutritional deficiency of that vitamin/nutrient and to promote health. The U.S. Food and Drug Administration determine RDA.

Red blood cell—A red blood cell that contains hemoglobin and transports oxygen and carbon dioxide in the bloodstream.

Retinoic acid—Vitamin A acid. A form of retinoic acid is the active ingredient in the medication Retin-A.

Rice syrup—Sweetener that is constituted by a complex carbohydrate; helps energy.

RNA—Ribonucleic acid, a complex protein found in plant and animal cells carrying coded genetic information from DNA — in the cell nucleus — to protein-producing cell structures called ribosomes, where these instructions are translated into the form of protein molecules — the basic components of all living tissue.

Royal jelly—A secretion from queen bee's nurse-workers that is rich in vitamins, minerals, enzymes and amino acids; it may be a natural antibiotic.

Salad—A Latin word for salt. Vegetables are excellent natural sources of sodium. Sodium supplementation is not generally needed (do not eat table salt). The body recognizes sodium from natural sources and also creates sodium from other salts. Potassium is an excellent salt substitute, as it reacts with hydrochloric acid in the stomach to produce sodium.

SAM-e—(S-adenosylemethionine) a naturally occurring compound in all living things which becomes depleted as we get older, or sick. It has many functions, but mainly helps joints in the body. It is also a mood stabilizer. Cannot be found in your diet.

Saturated fat—Fat that is solid at room temperature. Saturated fat is of animal origin, although some forms of it, such as coconut oil and palm oil, come from plants.

Sea vegetables—Dulse, hijiki, kelp, and others. Rich sources of protein, minerals and vitamins.

Serotonin—Brain neurotransmitter essential for relaxation, sleep, concentration, complacency and satiety.

Simple carbohydrate—A type of carbohydrate that is rapidly digested and absorbed into the bloodstream. Glucose, lactose and fructose are examples of simple carbohydrates.

SOD (Super-Oxide Dismutase)—An antioxidant enzyme, which helps neutralize, free radicals.

Sorbic acid—An organic acid used as a food preservative.

Spirulina—High-protein algae, rich in B vitamins and beta-carotene. Its high chlorophyll content helps digestion.

Sprouts—Sprouted seeds of alfalfa, red clover, mung bean, radish, sunflower, etc. Highly nutritious food, good source of protein, chlorophyll, Vitamins A, C, B and E, minerals and trace minerals.

Sublingual—Under the tongue.

Suma—An herb used since ancient times for energy. Promotes   hormonal balance.

Symptom—An indication of a bodily function or malfunction.

Thermogenesis—The body's ability to produce heat by burning calories. Stimulants, such as caffeine, increase thermogenesis. Normal body temperature is about 98.4 degrees, or anywhere from 96 degrees to 99 degrees Fahrenheit . Starving reduces temperature. Temperature below 94 degrees or above 110 degrees may cause death.

Tofu—is a cholesterol-free soybean food—contains complete protein (all essential amino acids).

Toxicity—The quality of being poisonous.

Toxin—A poison that impairs the health of the body.

Triglyceride—A compound consisting of three fatty acids plus glycerol. Triglycerides are the form in which fat is stored in the body; the primary type of lipid in the diet.

Triticale—A grain hybrid formed by crossing wheat and rye.

Unsaturated fat—Dietary fat that is liquid at room temperature. Unsaturated fat comes from vegetable sources and is a good source of essential fatty acids. Examples: flaxseed oil, sunflower oil, safflower oil and primrose oil.

Valerian Root—A powerful sedative herb used to treat stress, gas,   and cramps and to provide general pain relief.

Vinegar—A diluted and impure form of acetic acid, produced from or labeled brown rice, balsamic, apple cider, herb, raspberry, plum. Food preserver; helps digestion.

Virus—A minute disease-causing organism composed of a protein coat and a core of DNA and/or RNA. Because viruses are incapable of reproducing on their own, they must reproduce inside the cells of an infected host. Unlike bacteria, antibiotics do not affect viruses.

Vitamins—One type of approximately fifteen types of organic substances, essential in small quantities for life and health. Need to be supplied in the diet.

Water-soluble—Capable of dissolving in water.

Wheat germ and wheat germ oil—An embryo of the wheat berry, rich in B vitamins, protein, vitamin E and iron.

Wheat grass—A storehouse of vitamins, minerals, amino acids and enzymes used in diet supplementation. This powerful superfood cleanses and balances the body.

White blood cells—Blood cells that function in fighting infection and in wound repair.

Yeast—A type of a single-celled fungus. Certain types of yeast cause infection.

Yerba Mate—An herb used for energy and cleansing.

Yohimbe—An herb which purportedly aids in bodybuilding; some claim it has testosterone-stimulating capabilities.

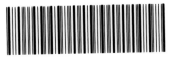